A Guide to Survivorship
for Women with Ovarian Cancer

A Johns Hopkins Press Health Book

Dr. F. J. Montz was Professor of Gynecology and Obstetrics, Surgery, and Oncology, The Johns Hopkins Hospital and Medical Institutions

Dr. Robert E. Bristow is Associate Professor of Gynecology and Obstetrics and Oncology, The Johns Hopkins Hospital and Medical Institutions

Paula J. Anastasia is Gynecologic-Oncology Clinical Nurse Specialist, Cedars-Sinai Medical Center

A Guide to

Survivorship

for Women with

Ovarian Cancer

F. J. Montz, M.D., K.M., FACOG, FACS
Robert E. Bristow, M.D., FACOG
with assistance from Paula J. Anastasia, R.N., M.N., O.C.N.

The Johns Hopkins University Press
BALTIMORE AND LONDON

Note to the reader. This book is not meant to substitute for medical care, and treatment should not be based solely on its contents. Instead, treatment must be developed in a dialogue between the individual and her physician. Our book has been written to help with that dialogue.

The Johns Hopkins University Press
2715 North Charles Street
Baltimore, Maryland 21218-4363
www.press.jhu.edu

Library of Congress Cataloging-in-Publication Data
Montz, Fredrick J.
    A guide to survivorship for women with ovarian cancer / F.J. Montz and Robert E. Bristow with assistance from Paula J. Anastasia.
        p.   cm.
    Includes index.
    ISBN 0-8018-8090-4 (hardcover : alk. paper) —
ISBN 0-8018-8091-2 (pbk. : alk. paper)
    1. Ovaries—Cancer—Popular works.   I. Bristow, Robert E.
II. Anastasia, Paula J.   III. Title.
    RC280.O8M66 2005
    616.99′465—dc22   2004019610

A catalog record for this book is available from the British Library.

Contents

Tables

Preface

A wish to write a "survivorship" guide for patients first arose when FJM (known as "Rick") was a fresh young faculty member in the late 1980s at the University of California–Los Angeles Center for Health Science. For the first time in his career Rick was caring for "his own patients." No longer were these women the responsibility of a public institution's clinic or the responsibility of an attending physician who allowed Rick to participate in the patient's care as needed. The patients looked to Rick as their personal physician, not only for cure and care but also for advice about how to get through the horrific experience that ovarian cancer can be.

The information that women with ovarian cancer desire and deserve was not readily available in a single place—a guide written for the patient, to be read, re-read, digested, and referred to as often as she wished. False starts in writing such a book followed. Most of the re-starts were motivated by patients who continued to express their wish for a guide they could turn to for everything they needed to know to relieve their intellectual, emotional, and physical uncertainties and suffering.

Years went by. Wonderful professional and personal relationships developed with two kindred-spirit professionals, Paula and Rob. We were all fortunate to serve as caregivers for many women, and the requests for a guide only amplified. Finally, the desire (or, more accurately, the *need*) to write this guide led us to pen the present volume. Our hope is that it will help a woman cope with the entire range of issues she will face in the daunting task of emerging on the other side of her encounter with ovarian cancer in one piece, an intact physical, intellectual, emotional, and spiritual human being.

Addendum: September 11, 2001, London
Death is an unwelcome partner that any oncologist must come to some degree of ease with, if the oncologist plans to continue to help women with ovarian cancer. But one never becomes "comfortable" with death. Today, in particular, I am uncomfortable realizing that, without any warning, thousands of my fellow Americans have been taken away from their loved ones. Being a frequent flyer and actually having flown previously on one of the flights that was highjacked, I think: "It could have been me." I have time to work on this manuscript simply because, instead of being home with my family, I am stranded in London, waiting for the FAA to lift the traffic stop so I can go home. An inconvenience, of course . . . but my family and I are alive.

Life is a sacred and limited commodity. We need to cherish it.

FJM

A Guide to Survivorship
for Women with Ovarian Cancer

Essential Concepts

Survivorship

Numerous philosophers have spent numerous hours discussing the "life well lived." Most of them would agree that the well-lived life is full of love, experiences, sharing, meaningful relationships, accomplishments, and giving to others. As we all progress along this journey, our attempts to live the "well-lived life" are threatened by different forces, both internal (for example, disease) and external (for example, social pressures) to ourselves. Ovarian cancer is only one of many such threats to the life well lived. The sense of betrayal by one's own body, the strain on relationships, and the physical toll that the disease and its treatments may inflict are some of the challenges that ovarian cancer presents to living life well. Yet it is the deliberate and conscious choice to live life well that allows us to truly *survive* as we navigate the uncertainties of human life. That is what this book is about: *survivorship* in the face of, in spite of, and through ovarian cancer.

What do we mean by *survivorship?* Of course, part of survivorship is just that: outliving the disease and being around long enough to live out one's natural life expectancy and die of something else. Do you have to be totally free of ovarian cancer to be a survivor? Absolutely not. Does being totally free of any viable cancer cell constitute survivorship? An equally forceful "No." Many women die from their ovarian cancer within a relatively short span of years or months, but they survive the experience, being mentally, emotionally, and, within certain limits, physically intact. Similarly, we have had numerous patients who have survived the disease, strictly speaking, but whose lives have been in shambles in all other respects. One woman, the one who actually dies from her cancer, is a survivor; the other, the one who lives many years or even decades "disease-free," isn't. What makes the difference?

The difference is in being in control as much as possible; being as "well," in all aspects of Wellness, as is possible; and finding joy and pleasure in ever having had a life well lived. Our mission, therefore, must be not to avoid death but to live life.

The Reality of Ovarian Cancer

Ovarian cancer can be viewed as three separate diseases. For some women, mainly those with early-stage disease and about 30 percent of women with advanced-stage disease, ovarian cancer is treated once and for all with an aggressive combination of surgery and chemotherapy. The disease is diagnosed, treated, goes away, and never comes back.

Unfortunately, for a small but significant second group of women, the initial treatments fail and the time from diagnosis to death is short—only months or little more than a year.

For most women, however, ovarian cancer is a chronic disease, one that is treated and goes into remission for a while and then returns, is re-treated, goes back into remission, and so on. Eventually, perhaps years or decades from the time of initial diagnosis, the patient will succumb to the disease or complications of its treatment. With this in mind, a greater emphasis is naturally placed on "what happens along the way," and the decisions made during these years or decades are enormously important.

Self-Determination

As we will emphasize repeatedly in this book, we firmly believe that the patient must be informed, as much as possible and as much as she desires, about the disease and about the treatment options and their side effects and outcomes. We are unshakably committed to patient *self-determination*. For a woman to determine what she wants, however, she must know what the choices are and what the results of such choices are. It is our obligation, as health care providers, to meet our patients "where they are," to help them to prioritize their wishes and desires, and to develop *individualized* goals and agendas, while presenting them with the information they need to make decisions about what they do or don't want. Only after all of these events have occurred can the well-informed patient have true self-determination.

Quality of Life

Another concept we will repeatedly focus on in this book is that of *quality of life*, often abbreviated as QOL. Simply defined, quality of life is how well a person feels about everything she is and everything that makes up her universe. It includes measurable factors such as the amount of pain or physical discomfort she is experiencing, but it is much, much more than that. Emotional, psychological, sexual, spiritual factors—all of them difficult to measure—are part of QOL. For many of our patients, the nausea, loss of hair, and pain cause less suffering than do certain fears about the future: what is going to happen to the patient's three-year-old daughter, her frail life partner for whom she is the primary caregiver, or her own soul.

Issues of quality of life must be addressed daily, if not minute by minute, when making decisions regarding treatments and other interventions. Many women are willing to trade a marked deterioration in their measurable QOL for a significant chance of a cure or a meaningful prolonging of life; few are willing to do the same for only a few additional months or weeks. Unfortunately, patients often are not informed that they have choices or that QOL can play a role in decision making. We believe that quality-of-life issues are the most important issues our patients face in exercising self-determination. One of our primary goals in our medical practice and in this book is to empower women to wrestle with these issues.

Chapter 1

What Is Ovarian Cancer?

Ovarian cancer is cancer that begins in the ovaries, which are important organs in the human female reproductive system. Normally functioning ovaries produce most of the human sex steroid hormones (*estrogen, progesterone,* and *androgens*); these substances control the start of puberty and sexual development and regulate the menstrual cycle. The ovaries are also the source of eggs (*oocytes*), which are released monthly (in the process of *ovulation*) in women of reproductive age. The ovaries of female babies already contain all the eggs they will ever have; as the girl matures, the hormones produced by her body cause the eggs to mature and to be released, ready for fertilization and growth into a fetus.

Most normal cells in the human body have a limited life span, which varies depending on their location in the body and the bodily functions they support. Normal cells are constantly being replaced. That is to say, in any normal tissue, some cells will be undergoing *cell suicide* (programmed cell death, or *apoptosis*), while new normal cells are being created to replace them. One hallmark of cancer is that more cancer cells are being produced than are undergoing suicide. This *reduction in the rate of programmed cell death* continues until ultimately normal cells are transformed into a *malignant tumor* (also called *cancerous growth*). Cancer cells not only divide and reproduce more rapidly than normal cells but also possess the capacity to spread to parts of the body located far away from the initial tumor (or *primary tumor*). When cancer cells spread in this fashion, the process is called *metastasis*. A *gynecologic malignancy* is a cancer that begins in the female reproductive organs. Ovarian cancer, in particular, represents the change of normal ovarian cells into a cancerous growth.

There are several different types of ovarian cancer. The most common type, *epithelial ovarian cancer*, is derived from the cells lining the surface (*epithelium*) of the ovary. Epithelial ovarian cancer is generally described in terms of two parameters. The first is what kind of subtype of cells is found, based on what the cells look like under the microscope (for example, *serous, mucinous*, or *endometrioid* cells). The second parameter used to describe epithelial ovarian cancer is called the *degree of differentiation*: are the cells well differentiated, moderately differentiated, or poorly differentiated? The degree of differentiation refers to how closely the cancer cells resemble normal, noncancerous cells. Well-differentiated cancer cells look very much like normal cells, while poorly differentiated cells don't resemble normal cells at all.

Other, less common, types of ovarian cancer include *germ cell tumors* and *sex-cord stromal tumors*, which begin in parts of the ovary other than the epithelium. These types of ovarian cancer are also known as *non-epithelial ovarian cancers*. Germ cell tumors arise from the egg-producing cells in the ovary; sex-cord stromal tumors come from the cells surrounding the egg-producing cells (the fibrous connective tissue, or supporting *stroma*).

For most women, the overall lifetime risk of developing ovarian cancer is small: less than 1 in 55. And ovarian cancer is not the most common gynecologic malignancy—endometrial cancer is. The sad truth, however, is that ovarian cancer is the number-one cause of deaths from a gynecologic malignancy. Approximately 25,400 U.S. women are diagnosed with ovarian cancer each year, and each year approximately 14,300 U.S. women die from this disease.

Although these numbers are saddening, it is important to put them into perspective. The most common cause of death for

American women isn't cancer at all; it is heart and blood vessel (cardiac and peripheral vascular) diseases. Almost one-third of all American women die from heart and blood vessel disease. That translates to 365,953 women a year! It has been proved and is widely accepted by the medical community that the most common causes of cardiovascular diseases are related to a person's lifestyle. Obesity, inactivity, high-fat diets, smoking—all increase the risk of developing these diseases.

The most common cause of cancer-related death for American women is also directly linked to lifestyle: lung cancer. More than 80,000 women each year in the United States are diagnosed with this disease, and 68,800 women die from lung cancer, most of them as a result of a cancer induced by cigarette smoking. Breast cancer is the most common cancer in American women, affecting 211,300 women each year. Fortunately, most women with breast cancer (almost 78%) survive this disease. Much of the success in breast cancer treatment is the result of early diagnosis, thanks to the wide implementation of breast self-examinations and mammograms. The other major cause of cancer morbidity in American women is colon cancer, a malignancy that is also strongly related to lifestyle. Cigarette smoking, a diet low in fruits and vegetables, and reduced levels of physical activity are associated with an increased risk of colon cancer. Colon cancer, too, can be diagnosed early, with stool occult (invisible) blood testing and colonoscopy (looking at the inside of the large intestine with a lighted telescope).

Risk Factors

We know what factors place a woman at higher-than-average risk of developing ovarian cancer. Those factors can be divided into the ones that are associated with "incessant ovulation" and the ones that are not. Table 1.1 lists these risk factors.

Incessant ovulation means that a woman releases at least one egg from her ovaries each month for a great many months. Early menarche (starting of menstruation), late menopause

Table 1.1. Risk Factors for Ovarian Cancer

Risk Factor	Increased Relative Risk*
Family history of ovarian cancer†	3 to 4 times
Older age	3 times
North American or European descent	2 to 5 times
Infertility	2 to 5 times
Nulligravid (no pregnancies)	2 to 3 times
High socioeconomic status	1.5 to 2 times
Late menopause	1.5 to 2 times
Early menarche	1.5 times

*Relative to the risk for women without the risk factor.
†In a first-degree relative (for example, a mother) or a second-degree relative (for example, an aunt).

(stopping of menstruation), few or no pregnancies, no breast-feeding, not using birth control pills (so-called oral contraceptives, or OCPs)—all increase the total number of ovulations in a woman's lifetime.

Many different theories have been proposed to explain why ovarian cancer develops. One theory is based on the idea that each time the ovary releases an egg (ovulation), the surface of the ovary ruptures (to release the egg). This process of rupture results in trauma to the surface of the ovary, which is then repaired by new ovarian surface cells. It is thought that repeated trauma and repair of this nature may result in an increased risk of ovarian cancer by incorporating an *oncogen* (an agent that contributes to cancer growth) into the healing cells or because a genetic mutation occurs during the repair process itself. This may be one reason that birth control pills, by decreasing the number of ovulations (and thus trauma), are partially protective against ovarian cancer.

Recent studies have demonstrated that repeated ovulation is not the only factor that plays an important role in the development of ovarian cancer. The balance between local (ovarian) concentrations of the sex steroid hormones estrogen and prog esterone, called the *hormonal milieu,* may also be important in the development of ovarian cancer. A shift in this balance from the normal progesterone-dominant hormonal milieu to one of relative progesterone deficiency has been associated with an increased risk of ovarian cancer. As we discuss below, progesterone, which inhibits ovulation, seems to be effective at decreasing (though not eliminating) the risk of ovarian cancer in more ways than one.

The most significant other risk factors for ovarian cancer are a family history of the disease and the associated genetic predisposition for developing the disease. A family history of ovarian cancer in a first-degree relative (a mother or a sister) or a second-degree relative (an aunt or a grandmother) makes a woman three or four times more likely to develop ovarian cancer. There are a number of potential genetic abnormalities that can lead to an increased risk for and eventual development of ovarian cancer. Most human cancers develop as a result of abnormalities (or *mutations*) in certain genes.

Genes are the functional units of heredity; each gene is located at a specific site on a chromosome. *Oncogenes* are genes that, when activated (by a mutation, for example), cause uncontrolled cell growth and produce a malignant tumor. Another group of genes, called *tumor suppressor genes,* normally function to prevent cancerous growths. When a tumor suppressor gene suffers a mutation, this normal preventive function is lost and a cancer develops. For example, the BRCA1 and BRCA2 genes, located on chromosomes 17 and 13, respectively, have been genetically linked to the development of both ovarian cancer and breast cancer. At most, however, only 15 percent of all ovarian cancers are the result of a genetic predisposition. Genetic predisposition may be associated with a similar increased risk of developing breast cancer. The genetic abnormalities are more common in women of eastern European Jewish descent (so-called Ashkenazi Jews). If the *lifetime risk* of ovarian cancer is defined as the possibility that a woman will develop ovarian cancer before living out her natural life of eighty-plus years, then in some women with these genes, the lifetime risk may be as high as 50 percent. Women such as these may benefit greatly by participating in some form of screening (screening is discussed later in this chapter).

In addition to family history and genetic predisposition, increasing age and certain demographic characteristics (high socioeconomic status, few pregnancies, infertility) are associated with an increased risk of ovarian cancer.

Prevention

We have identified the factors that put a woman at increased risk for developing ovarian cancer. Now we can discuss how a woman might decrease the risk. Obviously, we can't change who her parents were or when she naturally starts and stops menstruating. But there are things that can be done to decrease the number of ovulations over a woman's lifetime. It would probably be unreasonable to encourage women to become pregnant or breast-feed just to decrease their risk of ovarian cancer, because, as noted, the overall risk for the average woman is small. But is it unreasonable to encourage a woman to use OCPs as her means of birth control, particularly if there is a family history of ovarian cancer or a personal increased risk? We believe that using birth control pills is a reasonable approach to prevention in some women, and in fact we encourage women to consider this as an option.

There is growing evidence that taking exogenous progesterone (that is, progesterone not produced by the body), particularly in relatively high doses for short time intervals or lower doses for long time intervals, protects against ovarian cancer better than the approach of preventing ovulation alone. It appears that progesterone is effective at stimulating "suicide" by cells that have undergone the genetic and molecular changes that could lead to the development of ovarian cancer. This is an exciting finding, as it may offer an easy and low-risk way to decrease a woman's chance of developing ovarian cancer. We will want to see the results of thorough scientific testing before encouraging women to take progesterone as a means of preventing ovarian cancer.

In addition to progesterone, other agents (such as dimethyl-sulfoxide, known as DMSO) are presently being tested to determine whether they can decrease a woman's chance of developing ovarian cancer. At this time there are only limited preclinical human data to support the use of any of these additional agents. We anxiously await the results of ongoing clinical trials, as well as trials yet to be begun.

What about removing the ovaries as a way to protect against this frequently lethal disease? A procedure called *prophylactic oophorectomy* can be done, in which a woman's ovaries are removed even though the ovaries are apparently healthy. There are numerous problems with prophylactic oophorectomy in the woman who has no greater than average risk for ovarian cancer.

In most cases, prophylactic oophorectomy can be performed using minimally invasive surgical techniques. Minimally invasive surgery, also known as *laparoscopy,* involves the use of a small fiberoptic scope (the *laparoscope*) and small surgical instruments that are introduced into the abdominal cavity through three or four incisions that are 5 to 10 millimeters in size. The laparoscopic approach to prophylactic oophorectomy is associated with less pain and a shorter postoperative recovery time than the traditional approach via *laparotomy* (an incision in the abdomen). Nevertheless, even minimally invasive surgery is not entirely without risk. The chance of dying during surgery is 1 in 1,500, and 1 to 2 women out of 100 will have a major, life-threatening complication. The risk of having a major complication is about the same as the risk for the average woman of ever developing ovarian cancer. It just doesn't make sense in most cases to remove a woman's ovaries simply to prevent ovarian cancer.

The ovaries provide 95 percent of a woman's estrogen, so even for women who have a higher than 1 or 2 percent chance of developing ovarian cancer, there are significant concerns about what happens when the ovaries are removed. Estrogen is a hormone that a woman's body relies upon to keep nearly every organ working at its best. The potential problems with prophylactic oophorectomies are much greater for premenopausal women than for postmenopausal women. Beyond the simple but important quality-of-life side effects of an early (before the age of forty-five) surgical menopause, there is the fact that the average woman's life is shortened by removing her ovaries early if she doesn't take adequate doses of estrogen replacement.

Why shouldn't postmenopausal women who are at increased risk have prophylactic oophorectomies? The problem is that women who are at increased risk because of a genetic predisposition have about a 25 percent chance of developing ovarian cancer before they reach their midforties, and many of these same women are also at increased risk of developing breast cancer. Women who have a higher-than-average risk of developing breast cancer, and women who have had breast cancer, generally should not take hormone replacement therapy—therapy that is often desirable after removal of the ovaries. A woman who is facing these complex and difficult issues needs to consult a gynecologic oncologist who is well versed in the scientific data and who is a skilled and open communicator as well as expert in performing laparoscopic surgery (this surgery is described later in this chapter).

We strongly encourage any woman who is at increased risk of developing ovarian cancer because of personal variables (as described above), or because she has even one relative with verified ovarian cancer, to seek out the expertise of a gynecologic oncologist and discuss these complex issues.

Screening

In the United States, people who see a doctor for a regular checkup will be routinely screened for any number of diseases—breast cancer with mammography, cervical cancer with the Pap test, and prostate cancer with blood prostate-specific antigen determination (PSA), just to name a few. But routine screening is only possible if it is cost effective, and a cost-effective screening program for any specific disease is only possible under the following conditions: (1) the disease must be a common source of morbidity (illness) and mortality in the group to be screened; (2) there must be a pre-invasive or early invasive disease state that can be treated so as to prevent the development of either a crippling or lethal malignancy; and (3) there must be a method of screening that is easy and that poses little risk for the patient.

Ovarian cancer doesn't fulfill all of these requirements. The disease is not a *common* source of illness and death for U.S. women—not common enough to justify the expense of a broad-based screening program, in any case. For years the existence of a pre-invasive, or early, ovarian cancer remained unproven, and therefore no such "early disease" could be identified by a screening or early-detection tool. Similarly, until recently there were no reliable screening tools available. Fortunately, advances in screening for ovarian cancer have been made, and studies have shown that these new methods can identify early ovarian cancer.

The screening method for ovarian cancer uses a special type of ultrasound evaluation of the ovaries: *transvaginal ultrasound* with *color flow Doppler*. The ultrasound portion of this screening examination is used to evaluate the ovaries for any changes in volume (size) and morphology (shape) that may indicate an early ovarian cancer. Color flow Doppler evaluates the ovaries for changes in the pattern of blood flow to and within the ovaries. Certain characteristic changes in ovarian blood flow may be indicative of an early ovarian cancer. The combination of these two techniques can be used to pick up subtle cancerous changes in the ovaries and potentially allow for diagnosis and surgical removal before the disease has had a chance to spread. Before considering surgical removal of the ovaries for an abnormal finding on screening ultrasound, however, a woman should make sure that the ultrasound study has been reviewed by a radiologist with expertise in ovarian imaging and should consult with a gynecologic oncologist to discuss the results, the risks and benefits of surgery, and other options that may be appropriate (continued observation, for example).

But there is still the problem of determining which women are at *enough* of an increased risk to justify the expense of repeated ultrasounds and evaluation and subsequent management of changes that have produced no symptoms and are most likely nonmalignant. For example, a woman with no family history of ovarian cancer and limited personal risk factors is unlikely to develop ovarian cancer during the course of her lifetime. It is difficult to endorse routine screening in this case, because the expense and potential for personal anxiety associated with screening outweigh the small likelihood of detecting an early ovarian cancer. As with the issue of prophylactic oophorectomy, this issue requires the assessment of a woman's personal risk of developing ovarian cancer and her concerns regarding that risk. This sort of assessment is best completed by health care professionals skilled at risk determination and counseling.

We are fortunate to have such a group of individuals at the Johns Hopkins Hospital and Medical Institutions. These professionals work in concert with us in what is called the BOSS (Breast and Ovarian Surveillance Service), and we are all part of the Ovarian Cancer Network, a group of individuals who perform clinical trials investigating screening for and prevention of ovarian cancer. We are very liberal in referring to BOSS any of our patients who have questions regarding their individual risk of ovarian or breast cancer. If nothing else (and most frequently this is the case), patients are comforted when they find out that their risk for ovarian cancer is much lower than they had anticipated and that there is no need for intervention.

Symptoms and Diagnosis

One reason ovarian cancer can be a difficult disease to cure is that it often has spread extensively by the time it is diagnosed. Another reason is that the treatments do not work completely for everyone. But the fact that the disease so often has spread before it is diagnosed helps to illustrate the point that there are no *unique* symptoms and few *unique* findings upon examination or laboratory testing for ovarian cancer—there are no unique symptoms or findings that can lead a health care professional to make a definite diagnosis very early. The idea that ovarian cancer is a "silent killer" has recently been proved to be a myth, however. The vast majority of women with either early or late disease do have some presenting symptoms. (The term *presenting symptoms* is doctor-speak for whatever caused a person to seek medical attention in the first place—for example, a cough, fatigue, or pain.) Unfortunately, all too frequently, these symptoms are either ignored by the patient or inadequately evaluated by the woman's health care provider.

Almost one-third of women who are eventually diagnosed with ovarian cancer experienced their symptoms for more than six months before the diagnosis was made. *This is unacceptable.* We encourage women to visit their health care provider when new symptoms persist. And if a woman's health care provider doesn't evaluate the symptom to the woman's satisfaction, she needs to demand further evaluation or even get a new health care provider. You have no better health advocate than yourself, and you need to make sure that your concerns are addressed adequately.

The common presenting symptoms of ovarian cancer, as reported by women with this disease, are listed in Table 1.2. To a lesser or greater degree, they are present in all of us. Furthermore, these symptoms are associated with numerous other medical problems that are common in women in the age group in which ovarian cancer most frequently occurs—women in their sixties and seventies. Other such medical problems include stool habit changes (often as a result of medications or dietary changes) and diverticulitis (inflammation of the large intestine as a result of small hernias in its muscle wall).

These symptoms are quite common and often are just part of being middle-aged or older. That is why many women who develop these symptoms put off visiting a health care professional. And when a woman with these symptoms does see her health

Table 1.2. Presenting Symptoms of Ovarian Cancer

Symptom	Frequency (percent)
Increased abdominal size	61
Abdominal bloating	57
Fatigue	47
Abdominal pain	36
Indigestion	31
Frequent urination	27
Pelvic pain	26
Constipation	25
Incontinence of urine	24
Back pain	23
Pain with intercourse	17
Unable to eat normally	16
Palpable mass	14
Vaginal bleeding	13

Source: B. A. Goff et al., "Ovarian cancer diagnosis," Cancer 89 (2000): 2068–75.

care provider, it is difficult for the medical professional to determine how aggressive to be in attempting to find out exactly what is going on. Not uncommonly, there is no rush to find the source of the symptoms—and an additional delay occurs, this time brought about by the health care provider. The prudent medical professional will make sure that a patient is up to date in her screening tests for cancer of the cervix (Pap smear), breast (mammography), and colon (colonoscopy). For most women, this screening will include, in addition to a mammogram, a recent sigmoidoscopy or colonoscopy (looking inside the large intestine to see if there are any abnormal growths). A thorough pelvic examination is a critical but unfortunately often excluded part of these evaluations.

Based upon the degree of symptoms that a woman may have and her underlying risk of developing ovarian cancer, further investigations such as ultrasounds with color flow Doppler and other imaging studies (CT scan [computerized axial tomography] or MRI [magnetic resonance imaging]) may be warranted. We strongly feel, however, that little time should be spent performing multiple additional studies that are remarkably inaccurate and potentially expensive and that can lead to delays in diagnosis and treatment. We encourage our colleagues not to hesitate to perform a straightforward and generally easy procedure that can lead to making the definitive diagnosis in a relatively low-risk way: a diagnostic laparoscopy. We were taught early in our training that the prudent cancer surgeon doesn't let the abdominal wall stand between him or her and the diagnosis.

When a woman has symptoms that suggest a possible ovarian cancer and imaging studies do not provide a firm diagnosis, diagnostic laparoscopy may be the correct step to confirm or exclude the possibility of ovarian cancer. Because this procedure is minimally invasive, it can generally be performed as "same-day" surgery. Although general anesthesia is required, recuperation time is usually brief (1 to 2 weeks) and postoperative pain is not excessive. Before undergoing a diagnostic laparoscopy for a suspected ovarian cancer, however, a woman needs to have an extensive and informed discussion with her surgeon as to the plan of action if the surgery does reveal an early ovarian cancer. Will a biopsy be performed? Will the ovary be removed entirely? Will a hysterectomy be required? If ovarian cancer is discovered, will there be a gynecologic oncologist available to consult during the surgery? These are all appropriate questions, and a woman should be completely confident in her surgeons' ability to competently manage any and all of the possible findings at a diagnostic laparoscopy.

In this chapter we have described the current state of knowledge about risk factors for ovarian cancer as well as preventive measures and diagnostic tests for the disease. It is always preferable, but not always possible, to prevent disease. When a woman develops ovarian cancer, optimal treatment is based on the triad of (1) appropriate and aggressive surgery, (2) state-of-the-art chemotherapy, and (3) comprehensive care for the needs of the patient and the people who are important to her. In the chapters that follow, we discuss in detail these three approaches to treatment.

Chapter 2

Surgery

At first glance, surgery may seem to be a straightforward concept: a problem exists, and the person has an operation to fix it. In fact, however, surgery is a complex process beginning well before the actual operation and extending for some time after recovery. Surgery for ovarian cancer is no exception.

The specific tests ordered to diagnose ovarian cancer, the procedures performed to treat it, and even the manner in which the surgery is carried out may be different in different medical institutions and even among different surgeons, depending on the physician's experience and judgment. This chapter presents our view of the most important issues surrounding surgery for ovarian cancer as it stands today. We recognize that other health care providers may recommend approaches that are different from ours—and we want our readers to recognize this fact, too. Different approaches may be just as appropriate as our approaches. Furthermore, as technology continues to advance and more research is conducted, certain aspects of the treatment program described in this book will be refined, and some of the approaches described here may even become outdated.

Diagnostic Tests

When a woman visits a health care provider because she is experiencing symptoms, the health care provider will probably recommend a series of diagnostic tests to determine the cause of the symptoms. Ovarian cancer, as noted in Chapter 1, shares symptoms with other health problems such as diverticulitis. When a patient describes symptoms that could signal a number of different problems, the health care provider will create a mental list of possible diagnoses (this is called making a *differential diagnosis*). Tests are performed to rule out or confirm the diagnoses on the list. As test results become known, one of the potential diagnoses becomes most likely, and then further testing can focus intently on ruling out or confirming that specific diagnosis.

When tests such as ultrasounds, CT scans (computerized axial tomography), MRIs (magnetic resonance imaging), or diagnostic laparoscopy indicate that a woman has ovarian cancer, then surgery is nearly always performed to assess the nature of the cancer and treat the disease. (To assess the nature of the cancer, the surgeons stage the disease. *Staging* is the process of determining the stage of the tumor, which is determined by the location of the cancer, the size of the tumor, whether other parts of the body are affected, and the prognosis. The doctor can prescribe appropriate treatment once she or he knows the stage of the tumor.)

The symptoms of ovarian cancer can be nonspecific. In other words, as mentioned above, ovarian cancer shares many of the same presenting symptoms as other disease processes. Since those other diseases would require a different form of treatment, they must be identified or ruled out before a woman undergoes surgery for ovarian cancer. For example, the intestinal symptoms associated with diverticulitis may be confused with symptoms of ovarian cancer, but if a woman has diverticulitis, surgery for ovarian cancer will not help her diverticulitis, which is actually located in the colon. A mammogram is mandatory, and any findings must be followed up by appropriate further studies or biopsies. A colonoscopy is also mandatory. Colonoscopy may identify the true source of the patient's symptoms if they are not being caused by ovarian cancer, and it may also reveal any coexisting conditions that might require additional procedures at the time of surgery for ovarian cancer (for example, colonic polyps or colon cancer).

If the patient has a history or symptoms of upper gastrointestinal tract diseases such as peptic ulcer disease, we recommend that she also have an endoscopic evaluation of the esophagus, the stomach, and the upper small bowel. Specific studies to evaluate the drainage system of the liver, the gall bladder, and the pancreas (a test called *endoscopic retrograde cholangiopancreatography,* or ERCP) can be done if the doctor thinks the results might provide valuable information.

After all of these tests have been done and before we make a decision regarding surgery, we prefer to obtain a special type of a computerized tomography study, called a *three-dimensional (3-D) CT scan.* This study helps us to accomplish two goals: first, to make sure that there are no other potential causes of the symptoms (for example, pancreatic cancer or cancer of the small intestine) that would either preclude or remarkably change the surgical procedure; second, to determine how extensive the surgery needs to be and the patient's ability to tolerate the surgery. Once all of this important information has been assembled, we begin to discuss the surgery with our patient and prepare her for surgery.

Preoperative Preparation

There is a direct relationship between how healthy a person is when he or she undergoes surgery and the chance of recovering from surgery quickly and well. We think the picture of this "health" includes more than just having well-controlled diabetes or normal blood pressure. It also includes being emotionally and psychologically ready for what might happen. And the only way a person can be prepared, as the saying goes, is to be prewarned. Keeping this in mind, during the preoperative period we take however much time is needed to educate each patient, so that the patient will understand what is going to happen. At Johns

Hopkins we are fortunate in having a colleague who is gifted in patient education. She is a blessing!

Before surgery, the patient must have a chest X-ray, an electrocardiogram, and a wide array of blood tests. (These "pre-op" tests are done in addition to the tests mentioned above.) The patient is asked to visit her primary care provider for an overall examination and to make sure that any medical problems she has are being managed and are under control, if possible. Sometimes it is necessary to do special studies (a stress test or an echocardiogram) to determine how healthy her heart is, or to do pulmonary function tests to evaluate the health of her lungs. These tests help make sure there are no unknown risks to the patient in undergoing surgery.

In most cases the patient meets with the anesthesia team, who examine her and discuss the choices for anesthesia and postoperative pain management. And of course, before surgery, insurance company approval must be obtained, or an alternative method of payment must be verified, generally with the hospital's business office.

The preoperative visit with the surgical team is also very important. Generally the patient meets with the surgical team a day or so before the surgery. During this visit, the reason for surgery as well as the risks, benefits, and other options are reviewed. The "nuts and bolts" of the surgical procedure are described step by step for the patient. In other words, the surgeon will go through every possible contingency in a stepwise fashion and will explain what will happen for every possible finding: "If we find *this,* then we will do *this,*" and so on. The patient should feel free to ask questions about the different aspects of the planned procedure until she fully understands what is going to happen. It is the surgeon's responsibility to make recommendations for treatment that, according to standard medical practice, are in the best interests of the patient. However, the autonomy and wishes of the patient must always be respected as the ultimate factor that determines what and how much surgery is actually performed.

Because we cannot consult with the patient herself *during* the surgery, the pre-op visit is our opportunity to make sure that she and we are "on the same page" about what to do for every specific operative finding.

The evening before surgery, the patient must completely empty her bowel by going through a bowel preparation. Preparing the bowel for surgery usually involves a combination of taking oral cathartics (for example, magnesium citrate) and enemas. Antibiotics may also be given, to reduce the bacterial content in the colon and minimize the risk of contamination if bowel surgery is necessary. For reasons we explain below, we have been known to cancel a patient's surgery if, when we perform the examination under anesthesia in the operating room, we find an uncleared bowel. No one wants this outcome, but it is in the patient's own interests not to proceed under those circumstances.

Bowel preparation is essential if the surgeon needs to make an incision into the intestine or do a resection of (that is, remove) a segment of the intestine to remove all of the cancer. If ovarian cancer has spread to the bowel wall, then the surgeon may need to resect the involved portion of intestine and perform a *re-anastomosis,* hooking back together the tumor-free bowel on either side of the removed portion of intestine. A bowel preparation significantly increases the safety of this procedure by reducing the risk of infection following any intestinal surgery. (The inside of the intestine normally contains a large quantity of bacteria, and the bowel preparation reduces the bacterial content.)

Finally, the patient's nutritional state plays a major role in how she does in surgery. We are convinced of the value of preoperative nutritional support. Scientific research has shown that when a patient has had significant weight loss or is malnourished, preoperative calorie and essential element supplementation can decrease the risk of significant side effects and even death around the time of surgery. When we are first consulted by patients who have diagnostic findings suspicious for ovarian cancer, we automatically address the issue of nutrition. Occasionally we will go beyond prescribing oral supplementation (high-calorie, high-

protein meal plans) to prescribe a ten-day or longer period of intravenous (IV) nutrition before surgery. Only rarely do we delay
a patient's surgery to allow for the ten days of IV nutrition, although, in the patient's best interest, we have done so.

Postoperative care is described at the end of this chapter.

The Surgical Consent

Signing a surgical consent is more than a necessary medical-legal
formality. *It is the conclusion of a process* during which the individual who is to undergo the surgery is educated about the procedure that will be done, the goals of the surgical procedure, the
alternatives to undergoing surgery, and the complications that
can occur (this should include a thorough listing of both immediate and delayed complications or side effects). We strongly believe that if at all possible, the consent

~should be obtained by the senior operating surgeon;
~should be obtained a couple of days before the surgery; and
~should be obtained only after an extensive educational effort.

The consent form has two parts. The first part should describe the reason for surgery, the planned procedure, and any additional procedures that may be warranted depending on the operative findings. If the patient is not entirely comfortable with this
part of the consent, she may request that modifications be made
that more accurately reflect her wishes and priorities. The second
part of the informed consent should review the potential risks
and complications of the surgery. Signing the informed consent
does not mean that all of the proposed procedures will necessarily be performed, nor that all of the possible complications
described will occur. A patient's signature on the informed consent simply indicates that her surgeon has explained these aspects
of the surgery in sufficient detail so that the patient understands
and agrees to undergo the stated procedure or procedures.

If a nurse or a surgical assistant whom the patient may never
have met obtains the consent early on the morning of surgery,

immediately before the patient is to be taken into the operating room and while the patient is being poked and prodded in a half-naked state—this just doesn't allow the patient to make a clear-minded decision. In rare circumstances, in an acute situation, it may be necessary to obtain consent on the morning of surgery, so that the surgery can be done as soon as possible. In any case, the patient has the right to request that the senior surgeon review the above issues with her personally and to her satisfaction. Obtaining the informed consent for surgery is an essential and, in our view, nearly sacred *process*.

Fertility Preservation

Many women who are faced with surgery for ovarian cancer are concerned about preserving their ability to conceive a child and carry the child to delivery. The patient and her surgeon need to discuss this concern before surgery. Although the most common type of ovarian cancer, epithelial carcinoma (the type that originates from the cells on the surface of the ovary), does not usually occur at an age when women want to maintain fertility, it does sometimes occur in younger women. Certain other types of ovarian cancer (those that originate from the cells that produce the eggs) most often affect young women in their late teens. So, for many women, preserving fertility is a real concern.

For reproductive-aged women with a newly diagnosed ovarian cancer, women whose disease appears to be confined to a single ovary are the best candidates for fertility-preserving surgery. The primary goals of the surgical procedure for these women are to remove all of the disease that is visible to the naked eye and to perform a complete examination of the pelvis and abdomen to make sure the disease has not spread beyond the involved ovary. Often these two goals can be accomplished without removing both of the ovaries, both of the fallopian tubes, and the uterus. Although a woman who has had one tube and one ovary removed has a 10 to 15 percent reduction in fertility (from an 85% chance of pregnancy by the end of one year of reg-

ular unprotected sexual intercourse to a 70% chance), the likelihood of her conceiving are still very high.

In fertility-preserving surgery for ovarian cancer, only those
reproductive organs that are visibly involved with the cancer
should be removed, although any suspicious cysts or lumps on
an otherwise normal-appearing ovary must be biopsied. Whatever reproductive organs can be left should be left, because,
thanks to modern assisted-reproductive technology and surro-
gacy, many potential combinations of organs and donors can lead
to a pregnancy.

If chemotherapy is recommended, then for the woman who
still wishes to be able to conceive a child, it is important to do
what can done to protect the unreleased eggs (the eggs that have
not ovulated yet) that exist in the remaining ovary. Unreleased
eggs can usually be protected by temporarily stopping egg production (ovulation). Ovarian suppression can be accomplished
in several ways. Gonadotropin-releasing hormone agonists can
be used to suppress ovarian function, but because they suppress
ovarian steroid hormone production as well as egg production,
they are associated with menopausal-type symptoms. We prefer to use birth control pills (OCPs), which conserve egg production without causing menopausal symptoms; we start them
as soon as possible after the surgery has been completed and the
decision has been made for chemotherapy.

Initial Surgery

There are two essential and primary goals of initial ovarian cancer surgery. As we will state several times in this chapter, these
goals are most often met when the patient is cared for by an
ovarian cancer expert. The goals are, first, to remove all the cancer that is evident (this is called *cytoreductive* or *debulking* surgery) and, second, to do surgical staging. We will discuss staging
first and then debulking surgery. Then we will turn to the other
roles of surgery in the management of ovarian cancer.

Staging

Ovarian cancer is a surgically staged disease (see Table 2.1). This means that the stage of ovarian cancer can *only* be determined after a surgical procedure is performed, and this procedure includes taking biopsies of the sites where the disease is likely to have spread.

It is in the patient's best interest to have the surgical staging performed at the same time as the initial surgery for the management of the tumor that led to the surgery in the first place. Determining the stage of the cancer is of value both for determining treatment (specifically, whether a patient should receive chemotherapy and if so, how much) and for predicting outcome (the likelihood that the patient will outlive her disease). The value of performing such a procedure has been repeatedly demonstrated: nearly half of all women with ovarian cancer that is initially thought to be isolated to the ovaries are found, at the time of surgical staging, to have cancer in sites in addition to the ovaries. Three-quarters of these women have Stage III disease.

A question that is commonly asked is whether the surgical staging procedure can be completed laparoscopically. The answer is that, in the hands of a skilled laparoscopic gynecologic oncologist, it *can* be done. Perhaps a more important question, however, is whether it *should* be done that way. One of the concerns, and a great source of controversy among gynecologic surgeons, is whether rupturing an ovarian cancer that appears to be isolated to the ovary—a risk during laparoscopy—has a negative impact on cure. A second concern is whether there is an increased chance of "seeding" cancer cells into the tissue where the laparoscopic port sites have been placed. We believe that, when dealing with a disease as aggressive as ovarian cancer, it is better to err on the side of being conservative. If there is any concern whether a mass is malignant (based upon the presurgery imaging and blood work), we will do what we can to ensure that the mass is removed without rupture. If a colleague requests a consultation during a laparoscopic procedure on a patient who, after

Table 2.1. International Federation of Gynecology and Obstetrics (FIGO) Staging of Ovarian Cancer

Stage I Disease confined to one or both ovaries
    Stage IA Disease confined to one ovary
    Stage IB Disease confined to both ovaries
    Stage IC Stage IA or Stage IB with
                rupture of an ovarian cyst and/or
                cancer cells on the surface of the ovary and/or
                cancer cells in ascites fluid or peritoneal washings

Stage II Disease confined to the pelvis
    Stage IIA Disease involving the fallopian tubes and/or the
             uterus
    Stage IIB Disease involving other pelvic structures such as the
             pelvic colon, the bladder surface, or the pelvic
             peritoneum
    Stage IIC Stage IIA or Stage IIB with
             rupture of an ovarian cyst and/or
             cancer cells on the surface of the ovary and/or
             cancer cells in ascites fluid or peritoneal washings

Stage III Disease confined to the abdomen
    Stage IIIA Microscopic cancer cells in the abdominal cavity
             on biopsy
    Stage IIIB Abdominal disease 2 cm or less in diameter
    Stage IIIC Abdominal disease larger than 2 cm or spread to
             the pelvic, para-aortic, or inguinal lymph nodes

Stage IV Disease outside the abdomen (for example, in the lung or in the fluid around the lung) or involving the internal portion of the liver (parenchyma)

---

the ovary is removed, is diagnosed with an ovarian malignancy, we will decide whether we can perform the staging laparoscopically.

This decision is based upon numerous variables, including the patient's overall health, whether she has previously undergone surgery, has other ongoing medical problems, and so on. It is a highly individualized decision and one that we try to avoid making without first having a thorough discussion with the patient. One way to avoid this situation is for health care providers who are not gynecologic oncologists to refer their patients to a gynecologic oncologist *before surgery* when they have any concern that an underlying ovarian cancer might exist. Excellent-quality data support the belief that there is a four-to-five-times-better chance that a woman will have the correct staging procedure performed at the time of diagnosis of her ovarian cancer if the operating surgeon is a gynecologic oncologist than if the surgeon is either a general surgeon or a gynecologic surgeon.

Debulking

Debulking, or cytoreductive, surgery consists of removing as much of the tumor that has spread beyond the ovary as possible. This type of surgery is generally a major operation, performed through a vertical midline incision in the abdomen. In most cases, the cancerous tissue beyond the ovaries is visible to the naked eye, and the goal is to remove as much of this visible disease as is safe and technically feasible.

It is not a new belief that the amount of cancer that remains after the initial surgery is directly related to the probability that a woman will survive her ovarian cancer. In fact, the first articles establishing this outcome were published when the authors of this book were still in high school and junior high! Over the intervening almost three decades, however, the medical community has learned more about the relationship between cancer remaining after surgery, on the one hand, and survival, on the other.

It has been shown that, in general, if a woman's largest remaining tumor is 2 centimeters or less in diameter, there is a stepwise improvement in her chances of surviving with ovarian cancer for every bit smaller than 2 centimeters it is. (If there is a remaining tumor larger than 2 centimeters, it probably does not make much difference how much larger, because the future is not promising except, as discussed below, in those cases where *interval cytoreduction* or *debulking* can be performed.) The chance of cure increases as the tumor size under 2 centimeters decreases: 1 centimeter is better than 2 centimeters, small (*miliary*) disease is better than 1 centimeter, and no disease visible to the eye is best of all. By convention, *optimal cytoreductive* surgery indicates that *all individual tumor nodules larger than 1 centimeter* were removed. When *all visible tumor* is successfully removed, the surgery is referred to as *complete cytoreduction*.

Evidence from high-quality scientific studies increasingly supports the notion that there is absolutely nothing the doctor can influence, including choosing the type of chemotherapy, that affects a woman's chance of surviving her ovarian cancer as much as the quality of her initial surgery. If a gynecologic oncologist is the primary operating surgeon, the chance that a woman will have the best surgery possible (optimal or complete cytoreduction) is three times higher than if a surgeon who is not a gynecologic oncologist performs the surgery. Sadly, however, only between 30 and 50 percent of the women with ovarian cancer in any given geographic region will have optimal surgery. Data such as these make us plead with our nongynecologic oncology colleagues to refer any of their patients who have a significant chance of having an ovarian cancer to one of the nearly eight hundred gynecologic oncologists in the United States.

What is it about performing debulking surgery to remove large amounts of cancer that has such a remarkable effect on the chances that a woman will survive? It appears that multiple processes are involved. First, when the large volume of tumor has been removed, the patient is healthier overall, because she no longer has to "feed" the cancer. Feeding the cancer drains calories and other essential nutrients from her vital organs. She will also feel better, because she will no longer have the pressure and other *mass effects* of the tumors. Mass effects are the symptoms caused by a large ovarian tumor mass pressing on nearby organs, such as the bladder or the intestine. These may include urinary frequency or constipation, for example.

Second, it appears that when all the large tumor implants are removed, then any residual cancer cells are more likely to be killed by chemotherapy that follows surgery. This improved chance of killing the cells is thought to be a result of three things:

1. The remaining cancer cells grow more rapidly in response to removal of the large tumors. Because growing cancer cells are the only cells that can be killed by chemotherapy, this growth makes the remaining cells susceptible to chemotherapy.
2. The blood flow to the site of the cancer cells improves, which makes it easier to get both immune cells and anticancer drugs to the location where they are most needed.
3. Larger tumors are also more likely to contain cancer cells that have mutated to become insensitive to the killing effects of chemotherapy. It is thought that debulking surgery, by removing these drug-resistant cancer cells, can improve the effectiveness of chemotherapy.

Because the removal of any and all evident ovarian cancer is so important in a woman's odds of survival, it is equally important to do whatever is necessary, within reason, to achieve an optimal or complete cytoreductive surgical result. This often includes removing (in addition to the ovaries) the fallopian tubes and the uterus, a segment of the sigmoid colon and rectum, and parts of the large intestine and the small intestine. Thanks to advancements in surgical techniques and tools, *colostomy* (having the intestine drain into a bag outside the abdominal wall) is rarely necessary. The appendix, if it is present, is almost always removed.

Ovarian cancer commonly spreads to the *omentum*, an "apron" of fat hanging off the middle section of the large intestine (that is, the transverse colon). The omentum is frequently removed in its entirety to ensure removal of the maximal amount of cancer cells. Ovarian cancer can also spread to the peritoneal (or lining) surfaces of the abdomen and pelvis. Not uncommonly, a procedure termed *peritoneal stripping* will be performed, again to ensure removal of as many cancer cells as possible. Peritoneal stripping may be performed in the pelvis or the abdomen or both and is much like peeling the skin off an onion: only the outer surface lining is removed. Sometimes this procedure includes removing part of the top of the bladder.

Ovarian cancer also has a tendency to spread to the undersurface of the right side of the diaphragm, the muscle that separates the abdominal cavity (*peritoneal cavity*) from the chest (*pleural cavity*). Any tumor nodules on the diaphragm should be either excised (cut out) or destroyed using one of a variety of special instruments. We prefer to use what is called the *argon beam coagulator* (ABC) to vaporize the implanted nodules. Sometimes, however, it is necessary to excise part of the diaphragm to remove all of the tumor. This can usually be accomplished without an additional incision beyond the one that is already made on the abdomen. In select situations it is worthwhile to perform a *thoracoscopy* (placing a telescope through the diaphragm muscle and taking a look inside the chest) to make sure there are not any tumor nodules in the chest that need to be destroyed. Rarely, additional organs (gall bladder, spleen, liver, stomach) need to be removed in part or whole to successfully debulk a patient. If this is necessary, as long as it doesn't harm the patient, it should be done.

Neo-Adjuvant Chemotherapy and Interval Debulking Surgery

Although debulking surgery is the gold standard treatment for ovarian cancer, there are times when the surgery is not in the patient's best interest. Five to 8 percent of all women with advanced ovarian cancer are too sick to tolerate an aggressive surgery, or surgical removal is considered unsafe because imaging studies have shown their disease to be quite advanced or to be located in places that make surgical removal unsafe. Patients like this are probably best treated with what is called *neo-adjuvant chemotherapy with interval debulking surgery.*

In *neo-adjuvant chemotherapy,* the standard chemotherapy program is administered before attempting debulking surgery (rather than afterward). The term *interval debulking* refers to the fact that the cytoreductive surgery takes place after an interval of initial chemotherapy.

If the treatment plan involves neo-adjuvant chemotherapy with interval debulking, the first step is to collect a small amount of tissue, either through a needle or with a small incision (our preference), to confirm that the woman has ovarian cancer. If ovarian cancer is confirmed, then the patient receives about three cycles of standard chemotherapy (described in Chapter 3). During the two to three months of chemotherapy, aggressive attempts are undertaken to make the patient as strong as possible, using nutritional support to build her strength as well as medical therapy to treat any diseases she may have, such as hypertension, diabetes, or heart disease.

After she has had the three cycles of chemotherapy, the patient will have a repeat battery of imaging studies and blood tests. If the results demonstrate that there has been a remarkable response to the chemotherapy, and if the patient is deemed well enough to tolerate an attempt at interval debulking, then surgery will be undertaken. The goals at the time of interval debulking are the same as the goals of debulking surgery done as described above.

Scientists believe it is important to remove all the grossly evident cancer early in the chemotherapy treatment regimen to avoid having the patient develop *chemotherapy drug resistance*. In chemotherapy drug resistance, the cancer cells, being very adaptive, develop ways (often by mutating) to resist the killing effects of the chemotherapy. It has been proved that the more cancer cells there are, the larger the tumor nodules are; and the more cycles of chemotherapy that have been administered, the greater the chance of drug resistance. In neo-adjuvant chemotherapy with interval debulking, a race takes place between getting the patient healthy enough for surgery and getting the tumors small enough that they can be safely removed, on the one hand, and the cancer cells' ability to develop a way to resist the chemotherapy agents, on the other. No one knows exactly the best time to do interval cytoreduction in order to have the best chance of winning this race, or to achieve "the perfect balance," but after three to four cycles of chemotherapy seems to be the best time for most patients.

The Second-Look Procedure

Sixty to 70 percent of women who undergo the optimal initial debulking surgery followed by the optimal initial chemotherapy have no evidence of ovarian cancer on physical examination, imaging studies, and blood tests at the conclusion of their treatment program. Yet 60 percent of these women will see their cancer return. These tests, then, are not very accurate predictors of the future course of disease. Is there a more accurate way to determine what is "really" going on with women who are treated for ovarian cancer?

Numerous new tests *may* prove to be more sensitive than traditional CT scans and MRIs, but we do not yet know how good they are at identifying disease that does not show up on CT scans and MRIs. (The new tests include positron emission tomography [PET] scans—either linked with CT scans or not—that look at how special sugars are metabolized, and antibody studies that look for cells that produce little pieces of protein that are more likely than others to come from cancer cells.) One procedure, however, has been shown to be a remarkably accurate way of providing evidence of ovarian cancer and predicting the future: the second-look procedure. This procedure allows the surgeon to look inside the abdomen and obtain multiple *washings* (placing a saline solution in the abdomen, "washing" it around, and then collecting the fluid and examining it under a microscope for evidence of cancer cells) and biopsies of the abdominal lining and organs, collecting specimens that are examined by a pathologist to determine whether any cancer cells remain.

The second-look procedure can be done in two ways: either by laparoscopy or by making an abdominal incision. In the laparoscopic approach, the surgeon makes three or more small abdominal incisions (less than one-half to one and one-half inches in length), places small tubes called *ports* into the abdomen, and distends the peritoneal cavity with carbon dioxide (CO_2) gas so that long, thin *telescopes* can be placed inside the abdominal cavity. The "scope" is attached to a micro-television camera and the images are displayed on monitors in the operating room. Many procedures are completed as different types of instruments are placed into the abdominal cavity through the ports. The surgeon can peer inside the abdomen through the scope, can watch the images on the monitors, and can obtain washings and biopsies, all through the small incisions and the instruments inserted into the incisions. The other, and more traditional, way of doing a second-look procedure is through a large incision on the front of the abdomen (a laparotomy).

The advantage of the laparoscopic second look over the laparotomy is not that it is actually safer (causing fewer complications), though many cancer surgeons (including us) believe that it is. The real advantage is that women recover so much faster, usually staying in the hospital only overnight and being able to get back to their normal lives more quickly. Unfortunately, not all women may be candidates for laparoscopic second-look procedures, usually because they have extensive adhesions or scar tissue from the initial surgery. Nevertheless, approximately 80 to 85 percent of women who are candidates for second-look surgery can have this surgery performed using the laparoscopic approach.

Although it has been demonstrated again and again that nothing is more effective at discovering the status of a woman's ovarian cancer than a second-look procedure, the procedure remains controversial. Some physicians may not offer or even discuss second-look surgery with their patients who have ovarian cancer. When differences in recommendations exist, there is not necessarily an issue of right and wrong involved; the difference may be in philosophical approach. The majority of the controversy arises because second-look procedures have never been shown to improve the *cure rates* of ovarian cancer. This is because the prognosis is considered to have been set by the time a woman has completed her first surgery-chemotherapy regimen. There is growing evidence, however, that, although the woman's chance of having been cured has been determined by that time, what happens after the second look (consolidation chemotherapy, treatment with a salvage regimen, and so on—all discussed below) can make a difference in how *long* a woman lives a meaningful and productive life. More important, from our perspective, is the control she gains over her future.

Many women will choose to live their lives differently if they know they will inevitably die in a few years or even months, not decades, from their ovarian cancer. Women who find out that they have a negative second look and are in that subgroup of patients with the highest probability of being cured, however, may take a longer view of the future. *To us, the whole thing is about control and knowledge when making decisions.* We want our patients to know as much as they can. Therefore we encourage our patients to consider undergoing a second-look procedure. Of course, as with every decision that has any degree of risk, the patient must assess her risks and benefits in deciding whether to have a second-look procedure; for an elderly or frail woman, for example, the knowledge is of little importance and the risk, though small, is still excessive. All of these factors must be taken into consideration, balancing the individual's desires and goals, the advisability of the procedure from a medical standpoint, and the recommendations of the treating physician.

Secondary Debulking

If the disease comes back, additional surgery may or may not be an option. It depends upon how long the disease has been gone and in how many places it has reappeared. The concept of operating again on women who have recurrent ovarian cancer is called *secondary debulking* or *secondary cytoreductive surgery.* As the name implies, the surgeon is attempting for the second (or third or fourth) time to remove the cancer. More information is available all the time to help doctors determine who might benefit from such an attempt. Like second-look surgery, however, the concept of secondary debulking is controversial, and recommendations regarding its use may vary from hospital to hospital and from surgeon to surgeon.

This type of procedure is often more difficult and riskier than the initial surgery, primarily for these three reasons:

1. scarring from the initial surgery makes the surgery more difficult for both surgeon and patient;
2. the recurrent disease may be more deeply embedded in tissues than the earlier tumors were; and
3. the patient may not be as physically fit as she was at the time of the initial debulking.

Between 12 and 25 percent of women who have secondary (or tertiary, and so forth) debulking surgery suffer a potentially life-threatening complication. It is because of the very real risk of such a complication that we must be able to predict as accurately as possible before surgery which patients are going to benefit from the operation. We use a few general criteria. The women who are more likely to benefit from secondary debulking than to suffer a complication from it are women who

~ have had a relatively long disease-free period (at least six months, but the longer the period the better);
~ have physical and radiographic findings that show an isolated, solitary lesion or two (three lesions at most); and
~ have the physical "reserve" and psychological strength to undergo further chemotherapy.

The procedure is not without risk. Recurrent ovarian cancer commonly involves the intestine, and a portion of the intestine may need to be removed (and the tumor-free ends reattached) in the course of secondary debulking. Because of the complexity of these operations, blood loss can occur and a transfusion may be necessary. In addition, healing of the wound is often complicated by infection, separation, or hernia. Some degree of bowel dysfunction is also common. This may take the form of

- ～*ileus,* a slow return of normal bowel function as a result of literally slow bowel (which is usually managed by resting the bowel—taking nothing by mouth—until the bowel has a chance to recover);
- ～*bowel obstruction,* a blockage of the flow of fluid and food through the bowel (a partial bowel obstruction may respond without surgery to a course of bowel rest with a draining tube through the nose or the abdominal wall into the stomach, along with fluids, antibiotics, and nutritional support, or it may require surgical correction—but see below); or
- ～*fistula,* in which a hole develops between the intestine and the abdominal or vaginal wall and fluid from inside the intestine drains out. (Fistulas sometimes heal spontaneously but may require additional surgery to repair the leak.)

Women who are able to have a successful secondary debulking (that is, one that is "optimal" or better as described earlier in this chapter) will have about twice the life expectancy of women who either do not undergo the debulking or are unable to have a successful procedure. This is why we strongly encourage our patients who are candidates for this treatment option to consider having this surgery.

Palliative Surgery

When ovarian cancer returns and is no longer responsive to further therapy, medical problems such as bowel obstruction often develop. These problems theoretically could be treated surgically. It has been shown, however, that with rare exceptions, under these circumstances the surgery is more likely to harm the woman than to eliminate the symptoms. Similarly, we know that trying to surgically repair a bowel obstruction when the end of life is near is more likely to shorten a women's life than to alleviate her suffering and prolong a meaningful existence.

One procedure that *is* often performed to improve the quality of life for women who have nausea and vomiting because of bowel obstruction is the placement of a *percutaneous gastrostomy* (PEG) tube. If the nausea and vomiting cannot be controlled with antinausea medications and IV fluids, then a PEG is placed in the woman's stomach by endoscopy. In this procedure, a long, thin camera tube is slipped into the stomach through the mouth.

A PEG tube, which drains the stomach directly through the anterior (front) abdominal wall, can significantly improve comfort. It allows the stomach and intestines to be drained, acting as an "overflow valve"; furthermore, there is no need for the patient to have a fixed tube between her stomach and her nose, and she will not have to vomit. The PEG also allows her to take in fluids—an action that we have found can be remarkably emotionally gratifying and physically satisfying for patients—without the fear that she will vomit the fluids back up in a few minutes.

Postoperative Care

There is a dominant view—in our opinion incorrect—that, to maximize healing and recovery, the postoperative patient should physically do as little as possible. Nothing could be further from the truth. We know that the sooner women become active, the less likely they are to suffer surgical side effects.

Surgical side effects include

~ infections;
~ blood clots in the large vessels in the legs or pelvis—and pulmonary emboli, which occur when the clots break off and go to the lungs;
~ bowel dysfunction; and
~ muscle loss and weakness.

There is a lot of truth to the saying "Use it or lose it," particularly when it has to do with muscle function and strength. We recommend that patients get up and out of bed as soon after surgery as they can. Of course, as our patients are finding their "land legs," it is important for someone to help them get in and out of the bed or chair and to serve as a support, if necessary, when they are walking. When patients go home, we allow them to do light lifting (less than twenty-five pounds), walk up and down stairs, get out to the store or religious services, and go on short auto or train rides.

Another inappropriate limitation, in our view, is the prohibition on showering and getting the wound wet. As with walking around, there needs to be someone on hand to help and offer support, as a precaution against falling. But there is little chance of harm coming to a patient by getting the wound wet. Remember, the body is 75 percent water, and it is water that is helping the healing process. Getting an incision wet, or an IV or central line wet, has never to our knowledge been shown to have any negative effect on healing. The wound itself is "closed" by 18 to 24 hours after the stitches or staples have been placed. For this reason, although the wound has many months to go before the area regains its maximal strength, it would be difficult to harm it just by letting warm, soapy water rinse over it. And oh how wonderful it feels to be clean after a couple of days in bed!

As you can see, we are generally liberal about what we allow our patients to do. We do encourage them to be reasonable about driving after surgery, however. Just as it is against the law to drive with a blood alcohol level of 0.08 percent, it is also against the law to drive with narcotic pain medications circulating in the bloodstream. Beyond the slowed reaction time and impaired judgment, what about the ability to quickly move that foot from the gas to the brake when a buffoon runs the stop light in front of you? "De-acceleration injuries" like those that occur in automobile accidents can damage abdominal wall wounds and lead to hernias in the incision. Therefore, we want our patients to wait to drive until they are off narcotic pain medications and can move their legs freely and without restriction when in the sitting position.

Chapter 6 of this book is devoted to the issue of nutrition. We strongly encourage the reader to take the time to go through that chapter. But several general comments about postoperative nutrition are appropriate here. For patients who have not had major bowel surgery, the only special recommendations we give are the following:

1. Stay well hydrated. There is a natural tendency to become dehydrated, particularly in the postoperative period. In and of itself, dehydration can lead to constipation. The rule of "eight, eight-ounce glasses of noncaffeinated drinks per day" is a good one.

2. Avoid greasy, fatty, and spicy foods. Recently a patient of ours ate a meal when she left the hospital that consisted of a raw onion salad with a spicy olive oil dressing. And she wondered why she ended up in the emergency department later that evening with a world-class upset stomach! Surgery leads to stress; this stress leads to subclinical (that which cannot be detected by a physical examination) irritation of the lining of the stomach (the gastric mucosa). That is one reason why all our patients receive anti-ulcer medication in the immediate postoperative period. No matter how tough one's stomach is normally, it is going to be more sensitive for a while after surgery. Be nice to it and give it soothing, relatively bland comfort foods.

3. Get lots of bulk in your diet. The intestine has been cleaned by the preoperative bowel prep. Now it has to be filled up again. But you want to fill it with food that is going to go through it at a fast enough pace and hold enough water so it won't bog down and you won't get constipated. Fresh fruits (nonacidic) and vegetables, whole-grain foods, and so on are the order of the day. Avoid the so-called BRAT foods (bananas, rice (white), apple sauce, and toast) that we have all used to control diarrhea in our children.

After surgery, most patients begin treatment with chemotherapy. That is the focus of our next two chapters.

Chapter 3

Chemotherapy

What is chemotherapy? The term means different things to different people. Literally, *chemotherapy* means using *chemicals* (chemo) as *treatment* (therapy). Whenever a chemical of any kind is used in treatment of any kind, that's chemotherapy. Treat a yeast infection with an antiyeast cream—that's chemotherapy. Take an antibiotic to treat acne—that's chemotherapy. Take hormone replacement therapy to alleviate hot flushes—that's chemotherapy. And so is taking Taxol and carboplatin as a treatment for ovarian cancer after surgery.

What we usually mean when we use the term *chemotherapy* in the context of treating ovarian cancer is the *use of drugs that are administered with the specific intent to kill cancer cells*. And that is how we use the term in this book. In this chapter we describe how chemotherapy is currently used in treating ovarian cancer.

Three notes before we begin. First, you may hear health care providers use the term *cytotoxic agent* when referring to chemotherapy; the terms are often used interchangeably. Second, many new drugs are under investigation and may ultimately prove effective at preventing cancer cells from growing; some of these drugs are discussed later in this chapter. We look forward to having even more effective drugs to use in treating our patients in the future. Third, as with surgery, there are many different types of chemotherapy and different ways to administer chemotherapy for ovarian cancer. What this chapter presents is the authors' philosophy on "best care" practices as they exist today. Subtle differences in the recommendations of different health care providers certainly exist; again, these are based on an individual's personal experience and on the results of ongoing research studies.

We discuss chemotherapy for epithelial ovarian cancer first. Treatments for non-epithelial cancer are discussed later in the chapter.

Optimal Chemotherapy

Although there is some controversy among experts about how to define the concept of *optimal chemotherapy* ("best chemotherapy"), nearly everyone agrees that it is a goal we should strive to reach. Simply stated, optimal chemotherapy is chemotherapy that is given at the dose that is *maximally effective* while *minimizing chemotherapy-related side effects* to avoid compromising the patient's health and general well-being. Unquestionably, this balance can be difficult to maintain.

If the scales are tipped one way or the other, it is often toward the side of maximal effectiveness, even if there is a real (but, it is hoped, transient) compromise in a patient's quality of life. Here, as with all decisions regarding ovarian cancer treatment, the woman with the disease needs to be actively involved with the decision making. Specifically, in the case of optimal chemotherapy, an individual may be willing to take the potential risk of receiving a lower, and potentially less effective, dose of chemotherapy if such a dose reduction means that the chemotherapy-related side effects are tolerable to her. Much of this chapter and all of Chapter 4 focus on the prevention and control of chemotherapy-related side effects. Without these efforts to prevent and control side effects, optimal chemotherapy is very difficult to tolerate.

How Chemotherapy Works

Though it is not quite this simple, chemotherapy can be understood as working in one of two ways. Chemotherapy either (1) directly kills or accelerates the death of a cancer cell or

(2) prevents the cancer cell from successfully replicating (duplicating). Most chemotherapeutic agents work against cancer through a combination of these two pathways, but one of the two pathways predominates in each agent.

To understand how chemotherapy works, we have to begin by recalling (from Chapter 1) how cancer cells are different from normal cells—that is, noncancerous cells. The differences are a matter of degree, but in general the greatest difference is that cancer cells are uncontrolled in three ways: how fast they replicate, how long they live, and where they grow.

All normal cells reproduce themselves at a rate in the healthy state that has been optimized over millions of years of evolution or as a result of divine creation (depending upon one's view). They grow at just the right pace to maintain the function of the organ or group of organs they are part of. A good example of this process occurs when the skin is injured: skin grows back (through the process of cell replication) at a rapid rate until the site of injury is healed. In some situations (such as when keloids [excessive scar tissue] occur) there is exuberant growth, and the scar is thicker than necessary for the integrity of the skin. But even in these instances, the growth doesn't extend beyond where the scar should be, and it generally doesn't interfere with function.

The problem with cancer cells is that they don't stop. *They keep replicating.* As noted above, to stop the cancer cells, we attempt to interfere with their ability to replicate; if they cannot replicate, they die. Or else we allow them to replicate but we cause them to live for a shorter time; they can't replicate as fast while they are dying. The latter process is called *apoptosis* or *programmed cell death* (or *cell suicide,* referred to in Chapter 1). One of the problems with cancer cells is that they live longer than normal cells; apoptosis attempts to change that situation.

The chemicals that interfere with the ability of a cell to replicate do so by interfering with the production of specific cell chemicals or structures needed for successful cell division. With regard to the chemicals that stimulate programmed cell death, scientists do not fully understand the complex process. It probably involves stimulating certain genes in the cell that were not functioning previously.

None of the chemotherapy agents we currently use are 100 percent specific in their effects. That is, not only cancer cells but also normal cells are affected by these chemicals. Chemotherapy produces side effects precisely because normal cells are also affected.

Chemotherapy for Epithelial Ovarian Cancer

Front-Line Chemotherapy

In any cancer treatment, front-line therapy is the first chemotherapy given. It is designed to eradicate any cancer cells remaining after surgery (if surgery has been performed) and to achieve a complete clinical remission. A *complete clinical remission* means that, after treatment, there is no evidence of detectable cancer based on physical examination, imaging studies (for example, CT scan [computer axial tomography] or MRI [magnetic resonance imaging]), or serum tumor markers such as CA-125. (Serum tumor markers are blood tests used to monitor the cancer, and CA-125 is a serum tumor marker used to monitor ovarian cancer.)

Front-line therapy for the epithelial ovarian cancers may vary slightly from hospital to hospital in the United States, as well as from country to country around the world, but there is general agreement about what constitutes standard front-line therapy. The present standard is a combination of two different chemicals: a *platinum drug* (either *cisplatin* or *carboplatin;* the latter is our preference for reasons discussed below) and *paclitaxel (Taxol)*. These drugs have consistently been demonstrated to be the most effective up-front combination. Medical science marches on, however, and there are ongoing investigations to determine if adding another drug (such as *topotecan*) or giving the chemotherapy by another route (such as directly into the abdominal cavity) can improve either the outcome or the *toxicity profile* (the side effects).

At the Johns Hopkins Hospital and Medical Institutions, our preferred procedure for the administration of the Taxol and carboplatin is the following.

Baseline Tests. Before the chemotherapy is administered, we draw blood from the patient to obtain a set of baseline laboratory studies: a complete blood count (CBC) with differential and platelet count, a full chemistry panel, and clotting studies. We also obtain a baseline CA-125 or other tumor-related markers and a baseline series of radiographs (usually a chest X-ray and a 3-D CT scan of the abdomen and pelvis). These studies are extremely important. We will compare them with laboratory and imaging study results after the chemotherapy has been administered, to determine whether the chemotherapy is working and is being tolerated.

Central Access Catheter. A central access catheter has certain advantages for patients receiving chemotherapy. Most central access catheters are *semipermanent,* meaning that the catheter will stay in place for the duration of chemotherapy and will be removed afterward. A central access catheter has a real advantage because it provides a dependable infusion site for chemotherapy and other treatments (such as medications and blood transfusions). Placing a central catheter requires a minor ("same-day") surgical procedure. Some maintenance is required, such as periodic injections of heparin, a blood thinner, to keep the line open. A daily low dose of oral blood thinner (Coumadin, 1 mg) may also be prescribed, as it has been shown to reduce the risk of blood clots, which can clog the line.

There are two main types of central access catheters: external and implanted ports. External catheters are just that—access ports with one end located outside of the body; these catheters eliminate the need to stick the skin each time medication is administered, blood is drawn, or the port is flushed with heparin. Because the external port lacks the protection of an overlying layer of skin, however, it must be carefully cared for each day, to prevent infection. External catheters are inserted either just under the collarbone (called a Hickman catheter) or in the forearm (called a PICC line, for peripherally inserted central catheter). Implanted ports have a reservoir that is entirely underneath the skin; they have the advantage of a lower infection risk but the disadvantage of requiring a needle stick each time the catheter is accessed for infusion.

Chemotherapy Schedule. Different chemotherapy drugs or combinations of drugs can be administered over different time intervals, in what is called the *chemotherapy schedule.* Most drugs or drug regimens used to treat ovarian cancer are given every three to four weeks. This amount of time allows the body's normal blood cells (red blood cells, white blood cells, and platelets) to recover from the effects of one treatment and be ready for the next one. For some patients, however, the drug may be administered weekly or even daily, depending on the drug dose. Whatever treatment interval is prescribed, it is important to try to stay on schedule as much as possible to maximize the cancer-killing ability of the chemotherapy. If the normal blood cells are slow to recover, the treatment may need to be delayed. A delay of a week or so will not have any meaningful impact on the effectiveness of chemotherapy; because of this, we will occasionally modify the treatment schedule by a week or so to allow our patients to participate in important personal, social, or professional events without having to deal with the immediate side effects of chemotherapy or other chemotherapy-related disruptions.

Although our plan generally is to administer six to eight cycles of chemotherapy if a women has had optimal cytoreductive surgery (see Chapter 2), after the third cycle we formally reassess how the patient is tolerating the treatment and what is happening to the cancer. This reassessment includes a complete laboratory and physical examination evaluation and, when it is

deemed valuable, a repeat series of imaging studies. The purpose of the reassessment is to make sure that the cancer is responding appropriately to the chemotherapy treatment. In rare
instances, the standard chemotherapy program of carboplatin
and Taxol may not kill the remaining cancer cells effectively. If
the imaging studies indicate that this is the case, then the treatment program may be modified by, for example, changing to a
different combination of drugs. For the small percentage of
women whose cytoreductive surgery was not optimal, we will
consider another attempt at debulking surgery. The decision
whether to recommend further surgery is based on these studies showing whether a patient has had an adequate response to
treatment. For a woman who has not had any cytoreductive surgery and is undergoing neo-adjuvant chemotherapy, we will use
the reassessment studies to determine whether an attempt at debulking should now be made.

The Day of Administration. The day of administration actually
starts the night before. We recommend that our patients eat
lightly the night before, choose nonspicy and nongreasy foods,
and avoid heavy foods (like large portions of meat). For patients
who have had difficulty with nausea during previous chemotherapy cycles, we start the antinausea medications the night before and continue them the next morning (please see Tables 4.5
and 4.6 in Chapter 4). We also strongly recommend that our patients take in lots of noncaffeinated and nonalcoholic fluids
(more than eight glasses in all) during the afternoon, evening,
and morning before the chemotherapy. We have found over the
years that a lot of the unpleasant feeling patients have the first
few days after chemo is due to dehydration as much as anything
else. They just don't want to push anything in after a dose of
chemotherapy, and therefore they naturally "prune out." Women
who "supersaturate" or "tank up" as much as possible before the
chemo really seem to do better.

Generally it takes about a half day to administer one cycle of
carboplatin ("carbo") and Taxol. After the laboratory results have

been checked and the pre-chemotherapy medications have been given, and the dosing of the chemotherapy has been triple-checked, the chemicals are administered. The carboplatin is given first, running in the line over about a half hour. This is followed by the Taxol, which is given over about a three-hour period. The administration of Taxol is done slowly to avoid an allergic reaction to either the Taxol or the fluid it is mixed in. If a patient has become anemic and needs a blood transfusion, we generally try to do this at the same session and will infuse the blood after the chemotherapy is "in" and we are satisfied that everything is going well.

When the vital signs are fine and any short-term side effects cleared up, the patient is ready to go home. Several of the medications that are given before chemotherapy (for example, Benadryl or Ativan) may cause drowsiness, so we strongly recommend that a friend or a family member drive the patient home after treatment.

All prescriptions must be filled before a patient goes home from her chemo infusion center. This is critical. Chapter 4 discusses the medications we prescribe.

After Chemotherapy. The majority of women experience most of the acute side effects of chemotherapy within the first few days after receiving the cytotoxic agents. In the time period immediately after treatment, usually about three to five days, some women have muscle aches and joint pains (Taxol in particular can cause these pains). Mild analgesics such as Tylenol or Aleve often provide effective relief for muscle aches. Most patients receiving chemotherapy experience some degree of fatigue after treatment. The fatigue may last from a couple of days to a week or more. This toxicity can be cumulative; in other words, the longer the treatment goes on, the more tired the patient is after each treatment. Once the entire treatment course is completed, it may take several months or more to recover fully from the effects of chemotherapy.

An unsettled stomach—but not nausea per se—affects most women in the first few days after this combination of chemotherapy. We strongly urge our patients to keep taking their prophylactic antinausea medications during this period. If a woman develops nausea or vomiting, we encourage her to take different medications, as discussed in Chapter 4. For the first couple of days after treatment, meals should be light, low in fat, and bland, just like the meals the night before and during chemotherapy. Many of our patients tell us that the complex carbohydrates (pasta, rice, potatoes, and bread) sit well on the stomach. We can't emphasize enough the importance of staying hydrated: drink, drink, drink! (Not alcohol or caffeine, however.)

The neuromuscular side effects that *all* of our patients have to a lesser or greater degree are generally the most bothersome. These side effects can be divided into those that are nonspecific (feeling tired or wiped out) and those that are specific (changes in any of the five senses, though touch, taste, and hearing are most commonly affected). We discuss these side effects in Chapter 4.

The other universal side effect from the Taxol chemotherapy is hair loss on the head. Some women also lose their eyelashes and eyebrows. Hair loss usually starts about three weeks after the first Taxol infusion. The hair generally starts to grow in again approximately four to six weeks after the last Taxol infusion.

Getting Ready for the Next Cycle. One of the most remarkable advances in chemotherapy is not the new drugs we use, but our ability to minimize the possibility of death from the chemotherapeutic agents. Doctors have learned how important it is to keep a close eye on a patient's blood counts and laboratory values to avoid life-threatening complications. We recommend that patients have blood drawn for a repeat set of tests about ten to fourteen days after every cycle of chemotherapy. And we repeat these same tests immediately before administering the next cycle of chemotherapy. CA-125 and any other potentially valuable tumor markers can be checked on a monthly basis, though many experts argue that they only need to be done at baseline and after the third and sixth cycles.

The day or two before (or even the day of) the next dose of chemotherapy, we meet with our patients. Often this visit takes place on the morning of a half-day chemotherapy treatment scheduled for the afternoon. We find these pre-chemotherapy visits very valuable. They give us an opportunity to ask our patients specific and focused questions, allow our patients to ask their own questions, and give us a chance to do an interval physical examination and write or rewrite needed prescriptions. We also like to use these moments to discuss again many of the important issues surrounding living life to the fullest during chemotherapy.

Consolidation Chemotherapy

Consolidation chemotherapy (discussed here) and *salvage chemotherapy* (discussed in the next section) are important concepts in the treatment of ovarian cancer. Chemotherapy that is given after the initial chemotherapy program has been completed and there is no clinical evidence of disease is called *consolidation chemotherapy* and can be viewed as an "insurance policy" against the cancer's recurring. For most oncologists, attaining this degree of certainty involves performing a second-look procedure, but some doctors administer consolidation chemotherapy to women who have not undergone a second look but who are apparently free of disease (as far as can be determined by physical examination, imaging studies, and blood tests).

The theory behind consolidation chemotherapy is this: we know that as many as 50 percent of women who have undergone optimal surgery and optimal chemotherapy and who have no evidence of disease (as described in the preceding paragraph) will have their disease come back. It comes back because there are hidden cancer cells that initially responded to the front-line chemotherapy but did not respond completely, probably because these cancer cells possess some degree of resistance to the chemotherapy that was first administered. The thinking goes that, by administering the same drugs but by a different regimen or method, or by giving different drugs by a different method (our preference), we will kill these residual cancer cells in some of the women who have so-called invisible persistent disease.

It is our obligation as doctors to tell our patients about the choices in treatment options available to them as well as the risks and benefits associated with those choices. We also believe we need to provide information to our patients about how strongly the scientific data support one choice or another. Only a small amount of data supports consolidation therapy, but we believe that the data are strong enough to justify offering consolidation chemotherapy to our patients who fulfill the criteria for this therapy. Two variables seem to influence a woman's decision about whether to receive consolidation chemotherapy: first, how severe or disruptive the side effects of the front-line chemotherapy were and, second, her general view of the world. If a woman feels a need for that insurance policy—if she is a "belt and suspenders" type of person—she is more likely to opt for consolidation therapy.

One approach to consolidation chemotherapy is to administer chemotherapy drugs intraperitoneally (directly into the abdomen). A doctor may decide to use both a different approach (giving the chemotherapy directly into the abdomen in the hope of getting maximal local dosage with adequate systemic dosing and decreased systemic toxicity) and different drugs (ones that we hope any residual, hidden, microscopic cells will not be resistant to, because they will not have "seen" these drugs before). Delivering chemotherapy into the peritoneal cavity requires a surgical procedure to "implant" an access port under the skin of the abdomen that can drain directly into the abdomen and pelvis. This peritoneal access port is often placed during the second-look surgery. Once the peritoneal access port is in place, chemotherapy drugs may be administered directly into the abdomen, usually at intervals of three to four weeks, for a total of three to six treatments.

We need to emphasize that there is significant controversy among experts about the merits of consolidation chemotherapy. We hope it is clear to the reader why we think there is value to this approach.

Salvage Chemotherapy

Salvage chemotherapy is quite different from consolidation chemotherapy. Salvage chemotherapy is administered either when the ovarian cancer has not gone away after treatment (the patient was never "disease-free") or when there is unequivocal evidence that, although at one time the patient may have been disease-free, the cancer has now come back. We know that a cure in either of these situations is unlikely, but meaningful prolongation of a productive life for many months or years is not an unreasonable goal. These different situations generally lead to different recommendations regarding treatment.

Salvage Therapy for a Woman Who Either Has Not Responded or Has Responded "Suboptimally" to Initial Treatment. We know that these patients, in general, unfortunately have the shortest life expectancy of any of our patients. Therefore issues of quality of life and how the patient wants to spend the limited amount of life she has left are of paramount importance. In a recent year, Rick had patients in this situation who selected each of these options: no treatment and hospice support only; aggressive second-line chemotherapy using an FDA-approved drug; and intense alternative treatments. Individuals made their decisions based on three factors: how ill they were (the sickest women generally chose no further treatment); whether there was an upcoming event that they were willing to do anything to witness (for example, the woman who chose aggressive second-line therapy because she wanted to do whatever was possible to attend her granddaughter's wedding nine months down the road); and whether, although they were not willing to do nothing, they were also not willing to deal with the inconvenience and toxicity of cytotoxic chemotherapy (such women chose alternative treatments).

Salvage Therapy for a Woman Who Had a Complete Response to the Initial Chemotherapy. An important question here is, How long did the complete response last? How to treat a woman when the disease comes back is directly related to how long the disease was gone. In general, the longer the disease was not evident (the *disease-free interval*), the more likely it is that we would recommend administering again the same drugs that were initially used.

Although there is no hard and fast rule, our opinion is that if a woman has been disease-free for more than a year and then the ovarian cancer returns, secondary cytoreductive surgery should be considered first, and then re-treatment with carboplatin and Taxol should be considered. Of course, if a woman has had significant persistent toxicity from the initial carbo-Taxol chemotherapy, we may be more hesitant to consider treating her with the same agents again. In that situation, or when the disease has recurred in a relatively short time interval (less than twelve months but more than six), we would again consider performing secondary cytoreductive surgery but would follow that with a different chemotherapeutic regimen.

There is no limit on how many different salvage regimens a patient can receive. But when a particular regimen has failed, it is important to reevaluate the patient's goals before another regimen is started. Sadly, the general rule is that the more different types of chemotherapy a patient has had, the more likely it is that she will have side effects from the chemotherapy and the less likely it is that her ovarian cancer will be cured.

Other Chemotherapy for Epithelial Ovarian Cancer

In addition to the cytotoxic agents, other drugs are used in treating women who have ovarian cancer. Although none of these approaches to treatment are considered front-line treatments in the conventional sense, many of them are of proven benefit; some others of them are only of potential—and as yet unproven—benefit.

Hormonal Therapy

For years, health care professionals have known that certain types of cancers respond to hormonal treatment, even when the cancer has spread. Rick distinctly remembers a case when he was a second-year medical student that demonstrated the effect of hormonal treatment. On Saturday mornings there was an optional course on clinical disease that involved the presentation of classic examples. One Saturday morning the students learned about a man who had developed metastatic prostate cancer. Because testosterone (the major hormone produced by the testicles) stimulates the growth of prostate cancer, the patient had undergone an orchiectomy (surgical removal of the testicles) to stop his production of testosterone. Following that treatment, his metastatic disease shrank remarkably and his pain was significantly relieved. Unfortunately, this response didn't last for more than a year or so, and at the time of the case presentation, he was receiving estrogen, which functionally worked as an "anti-testosterone." Again, his symptoms decreased and his lesions shrunk.

This case demonstrates a phenomenon that can occur with *hormonally responsive cancer* such as prostate, breast, endometrial, and ovarian epithelial: if you take away the hormone that acts to stimulate the cancer (sort of "fuel for the fire"), metastatic lesions may shrink. A similar effect can sometimes be obtained by giving an antitropic (*tropic* means "growth") hormone. In a simplified fashion, these phenomena explain why tamoxifen and Arimidex work as treatment for breast cancer and why select women with metastatic endometrial cancer can gain some even long-term control of their disease with the use of progesterones (working as anti-estrogens).

The unfortunate reality is that hormonal therapy only works for a small percentage of women with ovarian cancer. Only about 7 to 10 percent of women with ovarian cancer who receive hormonal therapy will have a measurable response. *Measurable response* is by convention defined as a 50 percent shrinkage in the size of the lesion, in two dimensions, lasting at least two months. Cures have never occurred with hormonal therapy.

The explanation for such a poor response rate is that as most ovarian cancers develop, the cancer cells lose their ability to respond to hormonal signals. Two types of ovarian cancer respond better than the other types to hormonal therapy: ovarian cancer that is well differentiated and endometrioid ovarian cancer. Well-differentiated and endometrioid type cancers are more likely to retain their ability to respond to hormonal signals and to be inhibited by the effects of hormonal therapy.

Although the majority of ovarian cancers will not be sensitive to hormonal therapy, in certain instances we think it is rational to attempt such a therapy. For women who have recurrent disease that is shown to express *hormonal receptors,* it is worthwhile to attempt hormonal therapy, in our opinion. Hormonal receptors might be thought of as "docking stations" in the ovarian cancer cells; they must be present for the hormones to have any effect on the cell's growth. We can predict with a fair degree of accuracy whether a woman with ovarian cancer will respond to hormonal therapy by doing specific studies (immunohistochemistry staining, or IHC) on cancer tissue. These studies measure the hormone receptors in cancer cells. It is always preferable to test tissue that is obtained as recently as possible, because a cancer may over time lose its receptors. Tissue to be tested for hormone receptor expression can be obtained at the time of secondary cytoreductive surgery or through a more limited biopsy of a recurrent tumor mass.

Despite our ability to predict response to hormonal therapy, we would still attempt to treat with hormones some women whose tests have shown that the cancer appears not to express the receptors. These might be women who haven't had their hormone receptors tested, for example, or women who wish to do something to continue to treat their disease but don't want to have much in the way of side effects. These women are more likely to have more mature (well-differentiated tumors) of the endometrioid variety.

Progesterone (usually given in pill form) is the hormonal therapy usually prescribed for ovarian cancer. The side effects from progesterone hormonal therapy include weight gain, leg cramping, oily skin and hair, mood changes, and headaches. Most women find that these side effects are minimal, except for weight gain, which may actually be welcomed. Other hormonal regimens, such as tamoxifen, Arimidex, and gonadotropin-releasing hormone agonists, are also used sometimes, although the scientific data supporting such use are limited at best.

Growth-Inhibiting Therapy

Ovarian cancer cells are well-oiled machines that are programmed to grow. But like all biologic "machines," they require an array of complex chemicals and mechanisms to keep them functioning. Part of the medical challenge of conquering cancer cells comes from the behavior of the cells: either they lack certain gene products to help regulate (restrain) their growth (as we discuss below, under gene therapy), or they produce chemicals stimulating the production of all the cellular resources the ovarian cancer cells need to continue their uninhibited growth.

It has been proposed, quite rationally, that if we could devise a way to disrupt only the chemicals that stimulate growth of the cancer cells, we could then focus our therapy directly on the cancer cells and avoid negative effects on healthy tissues. Numerous experimental efforts using this approach have been made, including inhibiting the growth of blood supply that the cancer needs (*anti-angiogenesis therapy*), stimulating the cell to undergo programmed cell death (*apoptosis*), and others. It is vital that the readers of this guide understand two essential points. First, these are great ideas, and a large number of remarkably bright and well-funded scientists are working on them. Second, nothing has been shown to work yet. We can only hope that in ten or fifteen years, when a subsequent edition of this guide is published, we will have lots of effective growth-inhibiting treatments to report.

Gene Therapy

The principle of gene therapy is similar to that of growth-inhibiting therapy. But rather than trying to change the way a cancer cell produces essential cell proteins that play a role in making the cell work, the goal in gene therapy is to replace an abnormal piece of DNA, which is making the cell behave like cancer, with a normal piece of DNA that will make the cell behave (again) like a normal cell. Cancer cells act they way they do because of their genes, so this may work!

For some reason, at the core of what makes a cancer cell a cancer cell is the fact that the cell has developed an abnormal "command and control" mechanism. The command and control mechanism of all of our cells is the DNA inside the nucleus of the cell. We inherit our DNA from our parents (half from Mom, half from Dad). Encoded in the DNA that we received via an egg and a sperm is all the intelligence that the cells of our body ever needed to grow and work. Some individuals inherit DNA (or genes) that makes their cells in a certain part of the body go haywire. For example, a mutation in the BRCA1 gene makes it much more likely that some breast cells will start to malfunction, stop behaving as they should, and get out of control—that is, become cancerous.

We know that all cancer cells have some degree of DNA or genetic perversion when compared to noncancerous cells. One of the incredible advances in our understanding of cancer has been the identification of a growing number of specific genetic abnormalities that are involved in specific cancer types. Theoretically, if we know what the genetic abnormality is, and we can fix that abnormality, we should be able to get the cancer cell to function normally again, right? Right. But, like everything involving diseases of the human body, it is not that easy. First there has to be a specific and identifiable genetic abnormality. Second, we must be able to produce the DNA or other genetic material that we want to replace the abnormal DNA with. And third, we must be able to find a way to get that replacement DNA into the cell.

Fortunately, quantum leaps are being made in all three of these steps. Unfortunately, though some of the studies have produced initially interesting results (particularly those that look at replacing a specific genetic abnormality related to the function of a cell regulator called p-53), more advanced studies have not demonstrated the effectiveness that was hoped for. But that doesn't mean that scientists are giving up. With continued improvement in the ability to identify abnormalities, produce replacement genes, and get the genes into the cells using safe viruses as the carriers, there is continued excitement in the cancer research community about effective gene therapy.

Antibody Therapy

Just as cancer cells are genetically different from normal cells, cancer cells can express different antigens (pieces of protein on the surface of the cell or elsewhere) than do noncancer cells. Antibodies are proteins that circulate in the blood system that can react with (or bind to) antigens. Antibodies are very specific in their ability to recognize a particular antigen, sort of like being able to identify one of your family members within the multitude of people attending a rock concert. If a cell produces an antigen, then, in theory at least, science can produce an antibody against that antigen. When the antigen and the antibody bind together, they form a complex that is recognized by the body's own hunter-killer cells (the white blood cells called *lymphocytes*). The lymphocytes kill the cells, and the dead cells are cleared from the body by one of the body's "garbage disposal systems" (the liver is cleared via the gastrointestinal [GI] tract, the kidney via the urine).

The problem with antibody therapy is that it will only work if the cell we want to kill produces a unique antigen that isn't found on the surface of normal cells. That is, we want to target the cancer cell but not the normal cell. And unfortunately, cancer cells and normal cells often produce the same antigens. To date, cancer-specific antigens have been elusive. Cancer cells do produce select antigens in higher concentrations than normal cells, however (for example, the antigen HER 2/neu and the p-53 antigens). If we administer an antibody against these antigens, all cells that have the antigens will be affected, but the cancer cells more than others and, it is hoped, to such an extent that they will be killed. Because other, noncancer cells also produce the antigens, some normal, noncancerous cells will be attacked, as well. It is this targeting of normal cells that leads to the side effects of antibody therapy.

The idea of anticancer specific antigen antibody therapy makes good sense, but to date the successes have been limited, for the reasons described above. We hope that as we learn more about what makes cancer cells different from normal cells, we will be able to find cancer-specific antigens that will allow antibody production and avoid systemic side effects. Although great strides are being made, antibody therapy that is effective for many people remains a hope for the future.

Immunotherapy

Immunotherapy is similar to antibody therapy, in that it employs the wonder that is the body's own ability to fight infection and anything that is foreign to itself. However, immunotherapy is essentially different. In antibody therapy, what's being identified is a specific piece of protein that, it is hoped, is unique to the cancer cell. Antibody therapy is akin to putting a big red light (the antibody) on top of the cancer cell's antigen, making it easier for the body's cancer-fighting immune cells (the hunter-killer lymphocytes) to find the antigen, even though the number of lymphocytes is not increased. In contrast, immunotherapy stimulates the body to increase the number of cancer-fighting immune cells, the hope being that by sheer numbers they will be able to find and eradicate the cancer cells.

In antibody therapy, the hunter-killer white blood cells (WBCs) attack cells that are identified as being "different," in this case because they have antibodies that are attached to specific antigens. In immunotherapy, the number of these hunter-killer cells is being increased. This can be done a couple of ways.

A patient's own WBC precursors (immature WBCs whose precise immune function has not yet been determined) can be harvested and then, in the laboratory, the precursors can be "expanded"—that is, grown—so that many more WBCs can be placed back into the patient. Or, the patient is given a drug to stimulate the production of the desired WBCs inside the patient's own body or to make the specific WBCs that are present more effective at killing cells. This is a simplification of the very complex realities of immunotherapy.

Just as with antibody therapy, immunotherapy must rely upon the ability of the WBCs to identify and kill cancer cells while not killing many (any!) normal cells. Otherwise, the therapy will have an intolerable rate of side effects. To date the two biggest problems with immunotherapy have been that it doesn't work for the majority of cancer types (specific melanomas and renal cancers being the exceptions) and that the side effects can be extremely toxic.

Continuing the comparison with antibody therapy, the hope is that we will be able to improve on immunotherapy so that we can grow or stimulate WBC hunter-killer cells that attack and destroy cancer cells only. It is probable that immunotherapy and antibody therapy will be used together for maximum effect. We are hopeful, though in a cautious way, about advancements in this arena of discovery and treatment.

Non-Epithelial Ovarian Cancers

For the most part in this chapter we have been addressing the use of chemotherapy in the management of epithelial ovarian cancers. There are numerous reasons for this focus. First, the epithelial cancers are by far the most common. Second, treatment of these cancers is relatively similar (front-line therapy with Taxol and a platinum drug). Third, many of the non-epithelial cancers (the *stromal tumors,* in particular) are not as responsive to chemotherapy and therefore are not as routinely treated with a standard regimen.

Even though the stromal tumors are not responsive, the ovarian cancers called *germ cell tumors,* which arise from the cells that are part of what is needed to develop the egg, are often exquisitely responsive to multi-agent chemotherapy. The ability to treat germ cell tumors has been a great advance over the last couple of decades. The germ cell malignancies are much more common in young women who wish to maintain their potential for childbearing. In the past, the most common germ cell malignancy, the dysgerminoma, generally would be treated with radiation therapy. The radiation treatment was often successful but at a cost: infertility. In contrast, multi-agent chemotherapy, though it has a potentially negative effect on fertility, does not always cause infertility. When investigations in the 1980s demonstrated that we could treat these tumors with the same degree of success by using multi-agent chemotherapy, a major step forward was taken in balancing treatment, on the one hand, and quality of life on the other.

Investigational Drugs and Clinical Trials

A large percentage of women who develop ovarian cancer will have recurrence of the disease following the appropriate aggressive initial treatments. Unfortunately, it is not likely that their cancer will be responsive to approved therapies. If they wish to undergo further attempts to control their cancer, they have available to them three general options: take treatments (usually chemotherapy) that are FDA approved but not approved as treatment for ovarian cancer; take substances (whether identified as medications or in other categories such as *herbal therapies*) that have not been proved (using traditional scientific standards for proof) to work for any cancer; or participate in an investigational trial (also called a clinical trial). It is this third alternative that we discuss in this section.

Each week we see women who have run out of approved options as treatment for their repeatedly recurrent ovarian cancer. Many of these women are looking for and willing to take nearly anything that has any real chance of meaningfully prolonging a functional life. We are impressed by how much information they possess and how deep their understanding of clinical trials often is.

Clinical trials are designed to determine, in a stepwise fashion, whether a potential treatment is as safe, effective, and "good" as previously approved therapies. The steps, commonly called *phases*, are used to describe what sort of study is being conducted and what the goals of that study are.

Phase I Trials

The purpose of a phase I trial is to determine how much of any particular treatment can be safely given. Phase I trials are also commonly called *dose-finding trials* or *toxicity trials* or *side-effect trials*. Although data about whether the treatment works will be collected, this is not the purpose of the study. Many, many treatments are investigated in phase I trials and shown to be so toxic that no further investigation is undertaken.

Phase II Trials

The purpose of a phase II trial is to determine whether a treatment works: to find out whether the cancer responds to treatment. There is no attempt to compare the treatment used in the study to any standard therapy currently in use. The trial is done simply to answer the question, Does the cancer respond? Yes or no?

Often the phase II trial will also seek to determine whether a specific dose of drug will work better than a higher or lower dose of the same drug. Again, no simultaneous comparison is made between the investigational therapy and any other treatment, although the response rates will be compared to the results of previous studies (referred to as *historical controls*). The investigating scientists will compare how many people treated with the phase II drug responded and how that response rate compares to historical information published about similar groups of individuals receiving different treatments. In those studies where different doses of the same drug are administered to different groups of individuals, the results from the different groups will be compared to determine which dose works the best (meaning that it has the ability to treat the cancer with acceptable side effects).

Studies often combine a phase I trial and a phase II trial in an attempt to economize. Although such a combined study does not, strictly speaking, follow the rules, it makes it possible for investigators to find out more rapidly whether a drug should be quickly brought into the front line of therapy.

Phase III Trials

Phase III clinical trials are considered to be the gold standard of investigation. (The gold standard is that level of scientific evidence against which all other studies are compared.) In these trials, different people who are identified as having the same disease are treated with different therapies. Patients are assigned randomly to different therapies. This means that after the person has agreed to participate in the trial, neither the investigator nor the patient-subject has any influence over which treatment the patient receives. Usually one of the treatments used is the current standard—that is, the treatment that has proved to be the best therapy for the disease.

When no standard therapy has been identified for the specific disease, then phase III trials may compare two or more nonstandard drugs. An example of this was the trial comparing Doxil and topotecan (topo) in women whose ovarian cancer had failed to respond to both Taxol and the platinum drugs. For women in this situation, there is no standard therapy, but there are many different choices. The goal of the Doxil-topo trial was to assess both response to and toxicity of the two drugs.

The phase III trial is also called a *randomized controlled trial* (RCT). Some individuals add the term *prospective* (*prospective randomized controlled trial*), implying that the trial is done in a forward data-collecting fashion. In other words, the data (for example, the likelihood of responding to treatment) are collected as the study happens in real time. In contrast, a retrospective study looks backward to collect the data (after all of the responses have occurred). Scientifically speaking, the quality of information provided by prospective studies is considered superior to that of retrospective studies. This is why phase III RCTs are considered the gold standard for determining the most appropriate treatment for a particular disease.

Phase IV Trials

Phase IV clinical trials are not part of the conventional trial schedule utilized by the National Cancer Institute (NCI) and other government and nonprofit funding agencies. These trials, which are commonly performed and underwritten by the for-profit pharmaceutical companies, are essentially investigations carried out *after* a treatment has been approved and has been demonstrated to be superior. Generally, phase IV trials are performed in an attempt to obtain more information about effectiveness and toxicity while doing a fair bit of marketing of the therapy to the health care professional. The phase IV trial holds little unseen risk or unproved benefit for the enrollee.

Enrolling in Clinical Trials

To participate in a clinical trial, a patient has to meet a strict set of qualifications, or inclusion criteria. These criteria usually have to do with the patient's performance status (overall health), disease status (initial diagnosis or recurrence), whether there is disease that can be measured (to accurately evaluate the effectiveness of the new treatment), and the number of previous treatments the patient has received. These strict inclusion criteria are set forth in order to make sure all the patients in a specific trial are as similar as possible, so that any improvement in outcome (that is, response) can be confidently attributed to the new treatment rather than to differences in the clinical characteristics of the individual patients.

Informed consent is a critical aspect of participating in clinical trials. Informed consent includes a discussion of the possible benefits of therapy, although in many cases these benefits will not be precisely known (getting information about the benefits is the reason for doing the trial in the first place!). A review of the possible side effects is also included in the informed consent, and again, these may not be precisely known. For example, one of the main objectives of a phase I trial is to determine the specific side effects of a new treatment when it is given at different doses.

"Response" Standards in Investigational Trials

We believe it is critical for a woman and those who care about her to understand what sort of response rates are being looked for in the clinical trial setting. For a person who is participating in a phase II trial, a positive response is defined as a 50 percent shrinkage in at least two dimensions of the tumor, with shrinkage lasting at least two months. Several issues must be stressed.

First, *50 percent shrinkage*. This means that the cancer has to be measurable in two dimensions. It can be measured by an imaging study (such as a CT scan or MRI) or a physical examination. Disease that shrinks 50 percent or more is considered responsive disease. Disease that does not shrink but also does not increase in size by more than 50 percent is considered stable disease. Disease that grows more than 50 percent is growing or nonresponsive disease.

Second, *shrinkage lasting at least two months*. Two months is not a long time for a response to last for a treatment to be considered successful. Whether two months is meaningful will depend upon what the patient does during that time, feels like during that time, and anticipates after the two months are up. For example, as of the writing of this book, Rick has been alive forty-six years or, said another way, 552 months. Two months is less than half of 1 percent of the time he has been alive. The longer he is alive, of course, the smaller the percentage of his life two months makes up. However, over the last two months he has watched his second son's varsity football team make it to the regional semifinal playoffs, seen his daughter play soccer (very well), played air-guitar to a Linkin Park song with his third son while driving with the top down on his car on the way home from Mass, watched his eldest son mature as a freshman at Brown, been emotionally and physically intimate with his life mate, Kate, published a couple of articles, operated a bunch, consulted on scores of patients with gynecologic cancers, spent a few days in Italia with his mom and dad, and so on. Hopefully the point is made: though two months isn't long as a percentage of his life, man oh man, you can have a lot of joy in sixty days.

Whether the investment in inconvenience and side effects is worth the potential for a two-month or longer prolongation of life is an extremely personal decision. Our goal is to make sure that our patients understand what's involved when they are making decisions about treatment. It is our patients' decision whether to participate.

Finally, *chance of response*. Most phase II trials are considered successful if they have response rates (as defined above) in the 15 to 25 percent range, which means that a phase II trial can still be considered successful if 75 to 85 percent of the patients don't have a 50 percent shrinkage of their cancer that lasts two months or more. These are not high response rates. But it is important to remember that most women participating in phase II studies are women who have been heavily and repeatedly treated. It all comes back to one's perspective.

For phase I trials, response rates are not the outcomes of interest—side effects and "tolerability" of the treatment are. In phase III trials, response rates are compared directly to the effectiveness of the standard or comparison treatment, so the response rate of the investigational treatment is interpreted within the context of the response rate of the standard therapy being evaluated simultaneously. For example, if the investigational treatment produced a response rate of just 12 percent, this might not seem like much, but if the response rate of the standard treatment was only 6 percent, the investigational therapy would have produced a 100 percent increase in response.

Why are certain treatments never studied? There are many reasons why some treatments are never investigated in a phase I,

II, III, or IV format: first, there may be no data from nonhuman trials to indicate that the treatment may work in humans; second, there may be data from nonhuman trials to indicate that the treatment may work in humans, but the trials may also have shown so much toxicity that it was clear humans could not take the treatment; and finally, it may be that no one is willing to pay for the study.

It happens often that no one is willing to pay for a study, and this phenomenon has little to do with science and everything to do with the business of medicine. If there is no profit to be made once the treatment is proved to work, no for-profit company is going to underwrite the trial. A nonprofit organization will underwrite the trial only if the disease is common enough to justify spending the limited and valuable resources needed to perform the trial. And, particularly with treatments that are widely used, relatively innocuous, and not regulated (such as many of the Eastern herbal therapies), the companies that make the products may not wish to have a product study take place, for fear that the study may prove that the product does *not* work. They may not want to find out.

The decision to participate in a clinical trial should be individualized, should be based on the overall risk-to-benefit ratio for an individual patient, and should be interpreted within the context of other, more standard, treatment options that may have a more predictable (although not necessarily higher) likelihood of benefit and known side effects. That being said, we consider that by participating in clinical trials, our patients can contribute in an important way to the advancement of medical science and have the potential of receiving an effective treatment for their disease in the process.

Chapter 4

The Side Effects of Chemotherapy

You don't choose how you're going to die, or when.
You can only decide how you're going to live. Now.
—*Joan Baez*

In the previous two chapters we described surgery and chemotherapy as treatments for women who have ovarian cancer. Our goal when we treat women with ovarian cancer is to remove all the disease with surgery, if possible, and treat any remaining disease and any microscopic cells with chemotherapy. The ideal goal is cure, with remission and increased survival time as alternative goals.

When we consider which chemotherapy regimen to recommend for our patients, the patient's quality of life is as important as the effectiveness of the treatment. If you're being treated for ovarian cancer, you should discuss with your doctor and nurse any side effects you experience, whether the side effect seems to be just a nuisance or a major health concern. To prevent or decrease complications that can interfere with day-to-day living or with long-term health, health care providers need to know about their patients' side effects.

Side effects from chemotherapy occur because the cytotoxic agents attack both the rapidly dividing cancer cells and normal cells (as discussed in Chapter 3). Most side effects (for example, low blood counts) are temporary, lasting only about two weeks after the chemotherapy treatment. Others (such as hair loss) resolve after the chemotherapy treatments have been completed. Rarely, but sometimes, side effects may be permanent; hearing loss and peripheral neuropathy are two examples (*peripheral neuropathy* is numbness in the fingers and hands or the toes and feet).

Every person reacts individually to chemotherapy, and she may or may not have side effects. Also, different chemotherapy agents cause different side effects. Symptoms of side effects may be mild and may not interfere with daily life or with the chemotherapy schedule. If side effects become severe, however, the patient may need to be hospitalized; in addition, chemo therapy may be interrupted or delayed, possibly but not necessarily interfering with treatment responses. Because each person responds differently to chemotherapy, your doctor and nurse will decide what is the best recommendation for your situation. You also need to know that these recommendations may vary depending on a particular hospital's policy or the health care provider's personal experience in managing side effects.

If side effects are recognized early, it is easier to prevent them in future treatments, to decrease their severity, and to decrease the risk of potential life-threatening complications. In this chapter, we discuss the most common side effects of chemotherapy as well as how to manage them.

Low White Blood Counts (Leukopenia)

As noted in Chapter 3, a complete blood count (CBC) will be done before each course of chemotherapy, to monitor the patient's response to the chemotherapy, including side effects. One of the potentially most serious side effects from chemotherapy is low white blood counts (WBCs), a condition called *leukopenia*. Because white blood cells help fight infection, a low WBC means the person is at greater than normal risk of infection. A low neutrophil count (*neutropenia*) is of special concern, because neutrophils in particular help fight infection. Many of the agents used in treating ovarian cancer cause white blood cell levels to

Table 4.1. Chemotherapy Used in Ovarian Cancer That
Increases the Risk for Low White Blood Cell Count

Carboplatin	Navelbine (vinorelbine)
Cytoxan (cyclophosphamide)	Taxol (paclitaxel)
Doxil (liposomal doxorubicin)	Taxotere (docetaxel)
Gemzar (gemcitabine)	VP-16 (etoposide)
Hycamtin (topotecan)	

decline (see Table 4.1). The risk of infection is generally greatest seven to ten days after chemotherapy is administered.

Just because the white blood counts are low does not mean
that the person has an infection or will get an infection. The doctor and the nurse will watch the patient's condition carefully for
any sign of infection, but the patient is her own closest monitor, and she should contact her health care provider if she has
any sign of infection. If you are receiving chemotherapy, you
need to be aware of the common symptoms of infection, including fever and chills (see Table 4.2). (*Symptoms* are what you
as the patient experience; *signs* are what the doctor finds on
examination.)

A decrease in the WBC is a temporary side effect of chemotherapy, generally lasting up to ten days; the WBC usually returns
to normal in three to four weeks. Some doctors obtain a complete
blood count for their patients ten to fourteen days after chemotherapy, to check when the *nadir* (lowest level) of the WBC occurs, so instructions or medications can be given if needed.

The WBC is rechecked before each next scheduled chemotherapy. Chemotherapy will not be given if the WBC is too low.
The doctor may postpone the chemotherapy treatment for a
week until the WBC returns to a safe level, or a medication may
be prescribed to help increase the WBC and neutrophil counts.
A medication called *Neupogen* is given by a daily injection in the
arm to increase the WBC. The doctor may also prescribe an antibiotic to prevent infection or to treat an existing infection.

Table 4.2. Common Symptoms of Infection

Fever of higher than 100.5°F
Redness, drainage, tenderness, or swelling (especially from
    wound or catheter site)
Sore throat with white patches on throat or tongue
Productive cough
Burning with urination

Patient Education for Infection Risk

1. Wash your hands often, and always after using the restroom, before eating, and when taking care of pets.
2. Bathe daily and keep yourself clean.
3. Brush your teeth at least twice a day.
4. Avoid large crowds and crowded rooms where infection may be spread. This is especially important between ten and fourteen days after each chemotherapy treatment, when you are at greatest risk of infection.
5. Avoid people who have infections (colds, flu, chicken pox, and so on).
6. Watch your diet. Foods (especially eggs and meats) should be completely cooked, and fruits and vegetables must be washed clean of bugs and pesticides (which are not good to consume any time).
7. If you are in a sexual relationship, talk with your doctor or nurse about any precautions you should take. If your WBCs are very low, you may be asked to refrain from oral sex or penile intercourse for a short time. Using a condom may be recommended to help prevent infection.

When to Call your Doctor or Nurse

1. If you have a temperature of 100.5°F or greater. If you have chills, please take your temperature.
2. If you have any other symptoms of infection, such as cough; sore throat; burning with urination; or redness, swelling, or drainage from a wound or the catheter site.

Low Red Blood Counts (Anemia)

A person with anemia is producing a smaller than normal number of red blood cells (RBCs). Women who have had surgery and are receiving chemotherapy or radiation therapy (see Chapter 5), or both, for ovarian cancer are at risk of developing anemia. We monitor our patients closely for anemia and other side effects of chemotherapy.

Some women are not aware that they are anemic, because the condition has developed gradually, over a period of time. Other women experience fatigue, the primary symptom of anemia. Fatigue occurs because oxygen levels in the blood are reduced. Oxygen is carried in the RBCs, and with anemia, the number of RBCs is reduced. Information on levels of RBC, hemoglobin (Hgb), and hematocrit (Hct) is provided by the complete blood count. (Hemoglobin and hematocrit are laboratory results that reflect essentially the same thing—the level of RBCs.)

A person with anemia may have other symptoms in addition to fatigue (see Table 4.3). Other symptoms of anemia include headache and the sensation of becoming lightheaded, dizzy, or short of breath or winded during physical activity. A woman who is being treated for ovarian cancer and experiences any of the symptoms of anemia should report these symptoms to her doctor or nurse.

Chemotherapy does not need to be postponed for medical reasons if a woman becomes anemic, although she may feel too tired or just not feel well enough to receive chemotherapy. For patients experiencing severe or prolonged anemia, additional treatment may be needed. In some cases, a medication called *erythropoietin* may be prescribed. This medication is given as a weekly injection to stimulate the body's bone marrow to produce more RBCs; it usually takes effect only after several weeks of treatment. If the level of RBCs is dangerously low, or if there isn't enough time to allow for erythropoietin to work (for example, if the patient is scheduled for a chemotherapy treatment session), then the doctor may recommend a blood transfusion. Although blood transfusions are generally safe, the decision to

Table 4.3. Symptoms of Anemia

Fatigue	Irritability
Dizziness	Decreased ability to concentrate
Headache	Indigestion
Shortness of breath with activity	Lack of appetite
Feeling of being cold	Paleness of skin

administer a transfusion is not made lightly. The risk of acquiring the human immunodeficiency virus (HIV) after transfusion of one unit of blood is 1 in 450,000, according to the Centers for Disease Control and Prevention.

Patient Education for Anemia

1. Report any symptoms of anemia to your doctor or nurse.
2. Prevent injury. If you are anemic, you may not heal as well or as quickly as you normally would.
3. If you are dizzy, change position slowly from sitting to standing. Do not drive if you feel dizzy.
4. Plan scheduled rest periods around activities or social outings.
5. Maintain proper nutrition. Drink more fluids than usual. Talk to your doctor about taking a multivitamin with or without iron supplements.
6. Your doctor may order erythropoietin (EPO) given by injection (usually weekly) for several months to help increase RBC production.
7. Your doctor may prescribe a blood transfusion if your RBC is very low or if your symptoms are getting worse.

Low Platelet Counts and Bleeding

Platelets are a component of the blood responsible for clotting. People who have a decreased platelet count (called *thrombocytopenia*) are at increased risk for excessive bleeding in the form of easy bruising after minor trauma or excessive blood loss from a minor cut. Chemotherapy and radiation are common causes of low platelets. The platelet count generally decreases between seven and fourteen days after administration of chemotherapy and may take two to six weeks to return to normal levels. The normal platelet count is 150,000–400,000/mm^3; if platelet levels remain below 100,000/mm^3 at the time chemotherapy is scheduled, chemotherapy generally will be delayed or the dose will be modified.

Patient Education for Bleeding

1. Report any excessive bleeding or bruises to your doctor or nurse.
2. Avoid activities that may increase your risk for injury: sports (such as roller skating or bike riding), tooth flossing, enemas, anal penetration, shaving with a disposable razor, walking barefoot.
3. Avoid elective procedures that may increase the risk for bleeding, such as dental cleaning and other dental procedures, placement of a PICC line or central catheter, a biopsy, acupuncture. (A PICC is a peripherally inserted central catheter; it is similar to a Hickman catheter, but in a PICC, the tubing extends from the arm instead of from under the collarbone.)
4. Prevent constipation and bearing down with bowel movements. Use stool softeners and laxatives as needed.
5. Avoid medications that increase your risk of bleeding, such as aspirin, ibuprofen, digoxin, Lasix, heparin, and Coumadin. Talk to your doctor or nurse before stopping or starting a new drug.
6. If there are repeated delays in your chemotherapy, your doctor may prescribe a medication given by daily injection to increase your platelet level so that chemotherapy can continue.
7. Your doctor may prescribe a platelet transfusion if you have signs of bleeding and your platelets remain at a low level.

Nausea and Vomiting

Chemotherapy-induced nausea and vomiting (CINV) may be mild, moderate, or severe. Not all chemotherapy agents cause nausea (see Table 4.4). The feeling of being queasy and unable to eat or drink can be unpleasant and can lead to physical problems like poor nutrition and poor hydration. The goal is to prevent CINV before it occurs.

The risks posed by prolonged CINV are dehydration and kidney problems. CINV may also decrease a woman's energy level, interfere with her ability to perform daily activities, and adversely affect her quality of life, intimacy, and socializing. If nausea or vomiting is not controlled and the patient needs to receive fluids intravenously, these fluids can be given in the doctor's office or the treatment center.

Different classes of treatment are used to treat different kinds of chemotherapy-induced nausea and vomiting (see Table 4.5). If you do not get relief from your antinausea medication, notify your doctor or nurse sooner rather than later, so another drug can be prescribed.

Anticipatory Nausea

Anticipatory nausea occurs when the patient feels sick or throws up *before* receiving chemotherapy. This is a learned response and is associated with remembering a previous incident of being sick after a chemotherapy treatment. Some patients say they feel sick to their stomach if they simply drive by the treatment center.

Table 4.4. Chemotherapy Used in Ovarian Cancer That Increases the Risk for Nausea and Vomiting

---

Cisplatin (also includes nausea delayed up to 4 days)
Cytoxan (delayed nausea can last several days) ·
Hexalen (altretamine)
Ifex (ifosfamide)
Administration of a combination of chemotherapy agents

Table 4.5. Medications for Chemotherapy-Induced Nausea and Vomiting (CINV)

Class	Common Side Effects	Uses
Benzodiazepines Ativan (lorazepam), Valium (diazepam)	sedation, confusion, amnesia	anticipatory nausea/ vomiting, anxiety
Phenothiazines Compazine (prochlorperazine), Phenergan (promethazine), Tigan (trimetho- benzamide)	sedation, confusion, involuntary muscle movements (can be prevented with Benadryl)	acute and delayed CINV
Benzamide Reglan (metoclopramide)	sedation, diarrhea, anxi- ety, involuntary muscle movements (can be prevented with Benadryl)	acute and delayed CINV
5-HT$_3$ Antagonists Anzemet (dolase- tron), Kytril (granisetron), Zofran (ondansetron)	headache, constipation, blurry vision with Zofran	acute CINV
Steroids Decadron (dexamethasone)	euphoria, insomnia, edema, facial flushing if given in IV quickly; may cause perineal burning	acute and delayed CINV
Antihistamines Benadryl (diphenhydramine)	sedation, dry mouth, dizziness; some patients have reported restlessness	delayed CINV
Butyrophenones Haldol (haloperi- dol), Inapsine (droperidol)	sedation, low blood pressure, involuntary muscle movements	delayed CINV

Table 4.5. *Continued*

Class	Common Side Effects	Uses
Cannabinoids Marinol (drona- binol, THC)	sedation, dizziness, euphoria, paranoia, dry mouth, visual changes	delayed CINV
Anticholinergic Scopalamine patch	sedation, dry mouth, restlessness, headache	anticipatory and delayed CINV
NK1 receptor antagonist Emend (aprepitant)	fatigue, constipation, diarrhea, hiccups	in combination with other anti-emetics for acute and delayed CINV

To avoid anticipatory nausea and vomiting, we recommend that the patient take an anti-anxiety medication such as loraze-pam (Ativan) thirty to sixty minutes before chemotherapy. As noted in Chapter 3, for patients who have had a particularly difficult time with nausea during previous chemotherapy cycles, we often recommend starting the antinausea medication the night before treatment and continuing it the morning of the infusion.

Acute CINV

This type of nausea and vomiting occurs within the first eight-een to twenty-four hours of receiving a chemotherapy treatment. The medications recommended for avoiding or alleviating acute CINV are in a new class of drugs, called *5-HT$_3$ antagonists,* that work to block the receptors in the brain that cause CINV. This class of drugs is most effective when taken the day of chemotherapy and as directed up to two days after chemotherapy.

Three different 5-HT$_3$ antagonists are used to treat acute CINV: dolasetron (Anzemet), granisetron (Kytril), and on-dansetron (Zofran). They are recommended for women receiv-ing chemotherapy drugs that cause moderate to severe CINV.

They can be given orally or intravenously at the same time chemotherapy is administered. They do not cause drowsiness but may have other side effects such as constipation or headache. Your doctor or nurse will discuss the side effects of the medications with you.

Delayed Nausea

Delayed nausea and vomiting occur eighteen to twenty-four hours after a chemotherapy treatment and can last up to four days. Cisplatin produces nausea more than the other chemotherapy agents, and the nausea is often delayed. Carboplatin may be substituted because women experience less CINV with this drug. However, carboplatin has the disadvantage of causing more severe decreases in the blood counts (WBC and platelets). Decisions about which cytotoxic agents to use are made for each individual depending on how she tolerates the chemotherapy.

Delayed nausea is a challenging side effect because the patient may stop taking the prescribed antinausea medications if she has no immediate nausea or vomiting, only to experience nausea three days later. Thus, we recommend that you take a medication for delayed nausea, even if you are not vomiting or feeling nauseated.

There are many choices for treating delayed CINV. For chemotherapy that causes moderate to severe CINV, prochlorperazine (Compazine) or metoclopramide (Reglan) are recommended every six hours in combination with a low-dose steroid such as dexamethasone (Decadron) given every twelve hours. The Compazine or Reglan is taken for four days after chemotherapy to prevent delayed nausea and vomiting (see Table 4.6).

No one standard treatment is recognized for delayed CINV, and different doctors and patients take different approaches to overcoming this side effect of chemotherapy. There are many options, so if one medication does not control delayed nausea and vomiting, another one can be started. Instead of switching to new medications for delayed CINV, some patients continue to take the medications they took in the acute setting—and that's

Table 4.6. Common Regimen for Delayed Chemotherapy-
Induced Nausea and Vomiting*

Do not take any medication unless approved by your doctor.

Compazine 10 mg every 6 hours for 4 days after chemotherapy
or
Reglan 10–30 mg every 6 hours for 4 days after chemotherapy

In addition to the above
Take Decadron 8 mg every 12 hours the first 2 days after
   chemotherapy.
Then decrease Decadron to 4 mg every 12 hours on the 3rd and
   4th day after chemotherapy.
Then decrease Decadron to one 4-mg tablet in the morning for
   5th and 6th days after chemotherapy to prevent withdrawal
   fatigue.

If nausea and/or vomiting persists, you may take Ativan 1 mg.
(If you have consecutive days of chemo, you may need to take
   medication for acute and delayed nausea.)

---

*Delayed nausea begins 18–24 hours after chemotherapy.

fine, as long as the symptoms are relieved. The side effects for
Compazine and Reglan include drowsiness, which is generally
not a side effect of the 5-HT$_3$ antagonists, but the 5-HT$_3$s are
significantly more expensive and have not proven to work any
better than Compazine or Reglan in treating delayed nausea.

Patient Education for Nausea and Vomiting

1. Take the prescribed antinausea medications for four days
   around the clock as directed by your doctor and nurse. If you
   do not understand the schedule for taking the medications or
   if you do not understand other aspects of how to take the
   medications, talk to your doctor or nurse.
2. Contact your doctor or nurse
   ~ if you are unable to eat or drink fluids due to uncontrolled
   nausea and vomiting,

~ if nausea and vomiting keep you from doing things you want to do, or

~ if you lose more than two pounds in one day.

3. Inform your doctor or nurse if you are having nausea and vomiting more than two times a day, if your urine is dark yellow, or if you are not urinating as often as you normally do. (Dark urine and infrequent urination are signs of dehydration.)

4. Eating and drinking are best done thirty to sixty minutes after taking antinausea medication. You may want to change your diet temporarily to bland foods (avoiding fatty, fried, or spicy foods).

5. Eat small, frequent meals. If you do not feel like eating one or two days after chemotherapy, be sure to increase fluids so you do not get dehydrated. In addition to fluids, try soups, Jello, popsicles, and sodium- and potassium-rich sports drinks such as Gatorade.

6. Reduce odors (hot foods, perfumes, chemicals) that can cause nausea.

7. If possible, have someone else cook your meals for you. If this is not possible, freeze several meals before chemotherapy so you can reheat them when you do not feel up to cooking.

8. Relaxation techniques, visualization tapes, and acupressure have helped patients control nausea. Discuss these alternative options with your nurse or social worker, who can provide instruction or videotapes or audiotapes for you and can point you in the right direction for more resources.

Constipation

There are many causes of constipation, and many women have irregular or hard bowel movements, or difficulty moving their bowels, even without a cancer diagnosis. When a woman is being treated for ovarian cancer, however, she is likely to develop constipation, for any of the following reasons:

1. She is taking in less fluid and fiber, often because of side effects from chemotherapy such as nausea or vomiting.
2. She does not move around as much as normal or get any exercise, because of surgery or fatigue.
3. A tumor or scar tissue (adhesions) is compressing the lumen (opening) of her bowel.
4. She is taking the chemotherapy agents Navelbine (vinorelbine), Taxol (paclitaxel), and topotecan (Hycamtin), which often cause constipation (see Table 4.7).
5. She is taking pain medications, antidepressants, diuretics, iron and calcium supplements, or the antinausea medication 5-HT$_3$ antagonists, which often cause constipation.

If there is any suspicion that a bowel obstruction is the cause of the constipation, contact your doctor or nurse immediately. Symptoms of a bowel obstruction include nausea and vomiting (especially after eating), inability to pass gas, increasing abdominal girth and discomfort, and constipation.

A regular bowel routine, dietary habits, activity level, and medications all play a role in bowel regularity. The goal is to maintain a regular schedule for bowel elimination, and if possible to prevent constipation from starting. See "Patient Education for Constipation" (below) for specific information on these four components of regularity.

If you become constipated, your doctor or nurse may recommend that you try one of the many preparations available to address this problem (see Table 4.8). These include bulk producers, saline laxatives, osmotic laxatives, detergent laxatives, and

Table 4.7. Chemotherapy Used in Ovarian Cancer That Increases the Risk for Constipation

Hexalen (altretamine)	Platinol (cisplatin)
Hycamtin (topotecan)	Taxol (paclitaxel)
Navelbine (vinorelbine)	

Table 4.8. Laxatives

Bisacodyl (Correctol, Dulcolax)
Docusate sodium (Colace)
Lactulose (Chronulac, Cephulac)
Magnesium citrate (Milk of Magnesia)
Methylcellulose (Citrucel)
Polycarbophil (FiberCon)
Polyethylene glycol (Miralax)
Psyllium (Fiberall, Metamucil)
Senna (Senokot, Ex-Lax)
Sodium phosphate (Fleet enema, Fleet Phospho-Soda)

stimulant-type laxatives. Many people without illness manage constipation using their own judgment with over-the-counter products such as Metamucil, milk of magnesia, Dulcolax, Senokot, and suppositories and enemas. Among these many products, most people find one that comfortably relieves occasional constipation. Table 4.9 describes one regimen recommended for treating constipation.

Here are some specific "dos and don'ts" about these preparations:

Bulk products, such as Metamucil, should be taken with large amounts of water. If you are not able to drink large volumes of water or fluid, the bulk products are not the best choice for you. In addition, although bulk products are effective at *keeping* individuals regular, once constipation has developed, especially if there has been no bowel movement for several days, a bulk product may add to the problem by bulking up the stool and making it more difficult to pass. (Bulk products are effective for individuals with loose stool, to help give it form.)

Stool softeners are used to soften the stool as it passes through the bowel. A softener alone may not effectively stimulate a bowel movement, however, so both a laxative and a softener should be used.

Stimulant-type laxatives, such as Dulcolax and Correctol, may

Table 4.9. Common Regimen to Treat Constipation

Do not take any medication unless approved by your doctor.

Senokot-S, take 2 pills at bedtime.

If more than 2 bowel movements occur the next day:
Reduce dose to one pill at bedtime.

If no bowel movement:
Increase Senokot-S to 4 pills at bedtime (or 2 pills in morning, 2 pills at night).

If bowel movement occurs:
Continue same routine.

If no bowel movement:
Increase Senokot-S to 6–8 pills at bedtime.

If still no bowel movement:
Call doctor or nurse and make sure there is no impaction.

If no impaction, add one of the following:
Dulcolax tablet (may cause cramping)
Lactulose or Miralax
Magnesium citrate

---

cause cramping, but they are effective. These agents are the most commonly prescribed medications for treating narcotic-medication-induced constipation.

Osmotic laxatives, such as lactulose, are made of synthetic sugar molecules. They stimulate a bowel movement by drawing fluid into the bowel as they pass into the colon undigested.

Enemas can be helpful for removing stool from the lower colon, but if constipation has been chronic or there has been no bowel movement for several days, it may be better to take an oral product, which can stimulate the entire bowel. Enemas should not be used by anyone with a low white blood count or thrombocytopenia (low platelet count), because with an enema there is a risk that rectal tissue may be injured, leading to infection or bleeding.

Patient Education for Constipation

1. Talk with your doctor or nurse about your regular bowel pattern and find out from them whether your treatment will increase your risk for constipation.
2. Increase your fluid intake to eight, eight-ounce glasses a day, if possible.
3. Eat foods high in fiber and bulk (bran, whole grains, legumes, fruits and vegetables).
4. Increase activity by walking (around the neighborhood, around the mall, and so on), joining a gym, or obtaining a referral to physical therapy for an exercise training program.
5. Follow your doctor's and nurse's recommendation for bowel routine. You may need to take a laxative or a stool softener (or both) daily, and you may need to increase the amount you take as time goes on.
6. If you are taking pain medications, you will need to increase the dose of laxatives with each increase in pain medications.
7. Try to move your bowels at the same time every day (for example, after breakfast).
8. Call your doctor or nurse if you have not had a bowel movement in three days, or if you have nausea and vomiting, inability to pass gas, abdominal pain, or abdominal distention.

Diarrhea

Diarrhea is defined as more than two loose bowel movements daily. It is not a common side effect for women with ovarian cancer or for women who are being treated for ovarian cancer, but diarrhea may become a problem for someone who has had surgery on the bowel, has received pelvic radiation, or is getting certain types of chemotherapy. The chemotherapy agents used in treating ovarian cancer that most commonly cause diarrhea are 5-FU (5-fluorouracil), Doxil (liposomal doxorubicin), and Xeloda (capecitabine) (see Table 4.10).

Diarrhea can be a sign of a *fecal impaction.* A fecal impaction

Table 4.10. Chemotherapy Used in Ovarian Cancer That
Increases the Risk for Diarrhea

5-FU (5-fluorouracil)
Doxil (liposomal doxorubicin)
Xeloda (capecitabine)

---

occurs when hard stool is unable to pass normally through the
rectum, and loose stool seeps around the stool mass, with "diarrhea" the result. In this situation, laxatives and stool softeners are the treatment of choice. A rectal examination can confirm a fecal impaction.

Other causes of diarrhea are lactose intolerance (intolerance
of dairy products) and other food intolerance. Lactose intolerance can be an inherited condition, or it can develop a result of
repeated infections or chemotherapy. Removing dairy products
from your diet or using lactase enzymes or drops may stop the
diarrhea.

Inflammatory bowel disease, anxiety, antibiotic use, and use
of antacids containing magnesium can also cause diarrhea. Diarrhea is sometimes an indication of a viral or bacterial infection,
especially if antidiarrhea medications do not control the stool
output. Signs of infection include fever, watery bowel movements, or stool that contains mucus or blood. A stool culture can
identify an infection.

Patient Education for Diarrhea

1. Inform your doctor or nurse if you have more than two loose
   stools a day for more than two days
2. Inform your doctor or nurse if you have a fever higher than
   100.5°F, and if your stool is watery or bloody, or it contains
   mucus.
3. Inform your doctor or nurse if you have decreased urine output, dizziness, weakness, or muscle cramps, which may be
   a sign of dehydration or loss of electrolytes.
4. Your doctor may recommend over-the-counter antidiarrhea

products such as Imodium or Pepto-Bismol. Talk with your doctor or nurse about what might be causing your diarrhea before you take any medications.

5. If your diarrhea does not decrease or clear up with over-the-counter products, your doctor may write a prescription for Lomotil, codeine, or Sandostatin.

6. If your diarrhea continues for more than four days while taking antidiarrhea medication, a stool culture should be performed to check for infection.

7. Avoid high-fiber foods, caffeine, spicy and greasy foods, citrus drinks, and fruit.

8. Maintain a low-residue diet until the diarrhea clears up. (A low-residue diet reduces the amount of stool that ultimately makes it to the colon and in that way reduces the overall amount of stool passed.) The BRAT diet is commonly used when someone has diarrhea (bananas, rice, applesauce, and toast).

9. Hydrate yourself with sports drinks that contain electrolytes, such as Gatorade. Other choices include Pedialyte, rice soups, and broth.

10. Keep the skin around the rectum clean and dry to avoid irritation. Vaseline and Tucks, both available without a prescription, may offer soothing relief.

Hair Loss (Alopecia)

Alopecia is the term for any loss of hair (the Greek word *alōpekia* means "loss of hair"). *Alopecia totalis* is the term used when a person loses all of his or her scalp hair; *alopecia universalis* refers to losing all of the hair from the body. Hair loss as a side effect of chemotherapy occurs because chemotherapy drugs attack rapidly dividing cells, including hair follicles.

Not all chemotherapy causes total hair loss; many agents cause only thinning of the hair, and some agents do not cause any hair loss at all (see Table 4.11). Approximately 15 to 20 percent of people undergoing chemotherapy will lose eyelashes,

Table 4.11. Chemotherapy Used in Ovarian Cancer That
Increases the Risk for Hair Loss

Cytoxan (cyclophosphamide)	Taxol (paclitaxel)
Hycamtin (topotecan)*	Taxotere (docetaxel)
Ifex (ifosfamide)	VP-16 (etoposide)

*Hair loss varies.

eyebrows, and underarm and pubic hair in addition to the hair
from the head. Although hair loss is usually asymptomatic, some
patients report feeling scalp discomfort before and during hair
shedding.

Generally hair loss occurs over a two-to-three-week period
after the start of chemotherapy. The hair begins to thin and fall
out in uneven patches or strands, as noticed on the pillow and
when washing hair. No treatments (such as ice caps or lotions)
have been shown to be effective in preventing alopecia if the
chemotherapy agent is known to cause hair loss. Infrequent
washing and brushing of hair will keep hair from falling out faster
but will not prevent it from falling out altogether. Hair regrowth
usually begins four to six weeks after the drug is discontinued.

The emotional impact of alopecia is often underestimated.
Hair loss can have a profound psychological impact on an individual—so profound that she refuses treatment. Even though
the hair will return, the loss of hair is a reminder of cancer.
Women with long hair are advised to cut it short before beginning chemotherapy, to decrease the psychological impact of loss.

Many hospitals and cancer centers offer support groups and
classes on beauty and body image. The American Cancer Society provides a class called "Look Good, Feel Better," which includes makeup and beauty hints. Shopping for wigs, scarves, or
hats before the hair loss is recommended.

Sun sensitivity is a concern for women with alopecia, so the
head and eyes should be protected: use sunscreen, cover your
head, and wear sunglasses. In the colder months, heat is lost

through the head; wearing a head covering, even indoors, can increase comfort.

Patient Education for Alopecia

1. Discuss with your doctor or nurse whether the prescribed chemotherapy will cause alopecia.
2. Select wigs, hats, and scarves before hair loss occurs.
3. Cut your hair short prior to hair loss, which usually begins about three weeks after receiving the first chemotherapy treatment.
4. Protect your head, eyes, and face from sun by using sunscreen, head coverings, and sunglasses.
5. Ask your doctor for a prescription for the wig, for insurance purposes. The prescription should read: "Hair prosthesis for chemotherapy-induced alopecia." Not all insurance companies will cover this expense, however.

Fatigue

Fatigue (lack of energy, feeling tired, wanting to sleep a lot) is one of the most common side effects of cancer and cancer treatment. Fatigue may be a symptom of the cancer. It may even be the symptom that brought the patient to visit a doctor in the first place, before cancer was diagnosed. Surgery causes fatigue, and healing and recovery can take weeks to months. When chemotherapy or radiation is added after the surgery, it's easy to see how fatigue can become overwhelming in the first month or two. Radiation also causes fatigue, generally by the third week of radiation treatment. Fatigue may last up to six months after radiation is completed. Chemotherapy has a cumulative effect, and fatigue may be constant until treatment is completed. For some patients, fatigue may last up to a year after completion of chemotherapy.

There are many other causes of fatigue in addition to the direct effects of illness and treatment. Lifestyle can play a role in fatigue, as can a large dose of daily responsibilities (such as employment, housework, caring for family, and financial concerns).

People who do not get enough sleep, as well as people who get too much sleep, often report not having any energy. Poor dietary habits and lack of adequate nutrition and hydration can easily cause a person to feel tired and weak. Too much exercise, and not enough rest for the muscles between workouts, can cause fatigue, and so can a lack of exercise and activity. For most people, increasing activity (within reason) is an excellent way to increase energy levels. If you are recovering from cancer and cancer treatment, we encourage you to maintain your daily routine as closely as possible. Keeping up your daily routine can reduce chronic feelings of fatigue. Even if you need to rest after showering and dressing, and even if you are moving more slowly than usual, activity will keep your circulation healthy and prevent your muscles from weakening. Some patients keep a journal so they can identify their energy patterns and plan their activities or social events around their fatigue.

Fatigue is difficult to measure and may not be thought of as an important symptom. One way to measure your fatigue is to gauge how it interferes with your life. Tell your doctor or nurse how fatigue is affecting your life. Use a numerical scale from 0 to 10 to describe your fatigue as it affects you daily, with 0 being no fatigue and 10 being the worst fatigue you can imagine or have ever experienced. Discuss how your feelings of fatigue affect your mood, your daily activities, your concentration, and your ability to work or care for yourself and your family. Your doctor and nurse will want to know if the fatigue came on suddenly, which may indicate a serious problem, or gradually, which is common with treatment-related fatigue. Medical causes of fatigue include anemia and electrolyte imbalances, which can be caused by dehydration, vomiting, and diarrhea. These two conditions can be identified through a routine blood test and can be treated. Depression and pain can also cause symptoms of fatigue.

Patient Education for Fatigue

1. Tell your doctor and nurse how fatigue is interfering with your lifestyle and activities of daily living.

2. Rate your fatigue on a scale of 0 to 10, with 0 meaning no fatigue, and 10 meaning severe fatigue.
3. Keep a journal of your fatigue as it relates to treatment and activity.
4. Report any factors that appear to be related to your fatigue, such as headache, feeling cold, feeling dizzy, or becoming short of breath with activity. These are symptoms of anemia.
5. Discuss the cause of your fatigue with your doctor or nurse. Unless there is a reason for you not to increase your activity level, doing so may help to decrease feelings of fatigue. Walk around the house or walk around the block. Once you can walk this far, increase your walking time by ten minutes each week.
6. Maintain a balanced and healthy diet, including eight, eight-ounce glasses of fluid a day and a variety of foods providing protein and carbohydrates, as well as fruits and vegetables.
7. Plan rest periods or a short nap around fatigue, or before a social outing.

Peripheral Neuropathy

Peripheral neuropathy is a side effect that may result from receiving specific chemotherapy agents, such as cisplatin and Taxol (see Table 4.12). Sensory nerves (related to the sense of touch), motor nerves (related to movement and muscle tone), and the autonomic nerves (such as those in the intestine, related to involuntary movement such as digestion) are the peripheral nerves (the nerves outside the brain) that may be damaged by chemotherapy. Patients who have a history of diabetes, alcohol abuse, or vitamin deficiency are at greatest risk for peripheral neuropathy.

Peripheral neuropathy in chemotherapy usually affects the peripheral nerves in the fingers, hands, toes, and feet. Many patients describe the sensation as a tingling, numbness, burning, or feeling of "pins and needles" in the fingers or toes, or both. The pattern is generally called "stocking-glove" because the sensation usually does not go above the ankles (stocking) or wrist

Table 4.12. Chemotherapy Used in Ovarian Cancer That
Increases the Risk for Peripheral Neuropathy

Hexalen (altretamine)	Taxol (paclitaxel)
Navelbine (vinorelbine)*	thalidomide
Platinol (cisplatin)	

*To a lesser degree than the others.

(glove). Another symptom of peripheral nerve damage is weakness in the arms; this weakness may cause the person to drop things or have difficulty buttoning shirts, for example. Walking may be uncoordinated, and simple tasks such as driving may be difficult because the leg and the foot feel heavy.

Peripheral neuropathy is not life threatening, but it can affect an individual's quality of life. In most cases the neuropathy is temporary, although cisplatin can result in delayed and sometimes permanent neuropathy. Some women with cisplatin-induced neuropathy may not experience the onset of symptoms until three to twelve months after the treatment has been completed. Cisplatin may have a cumulative effect, however, and the neuropathy may get worse with each treatment. It is important to report any symptoms of peripheral neuropathy to your doctor or nurse.

Patient Education for Peripheral Neuropathy

1. Inform your doctor or nurse if you experience any numbness or tingling in your fingers or toes. Let your doctor or nurse know if symptoms get worse with each chemotherapy treatment.
2. Maintain a safe environment:
   ～ Wear shoes that do not easily slip off and do not have elevated heels.
   ～ Turn the light on before entering a room.
   ～ Use handrails and a cane for assistance with walking.
   ～ Floors should be nonskid and rugs should have a nonslip backing.

~ Use rubber gloves to wash dishes and pot holders to handle hot items.

~ Use gloves for gardening.

3. Your doctor or nurse may recommend vitamin B supplements (100 mg two to three times a day) or glutamine powder supplements (10 grams three times a day for five days the week of chemotherapy), or both, at the start of chemotherapy.

4. Massage and range-of-motion exercises (for example, opening and closing hands) may help with circulation in the affected area. Wearing socks and gloves may give some relief.

5. Apply ice or soak your hands or feet in cool or warm water for temporary relief.

6. Talk with your doctor about taking medications that may decrease the effects of the burning or tingling:

~ non-narcotic analgesics

~ narcotic analgesics

~ corticosteroids

~ anticonvulsants (gabapentin [Neurontin])

~ tricyclic antidepressants (amitriptyline)

~ Emla, or capsaicin cream

7. Talk with your doctor or nurse about complementary or integrative therapies that may be helpful in reducing the symptoms:

~ transcutaneous electric nerve stimulation (TENS)

~ acupuncture or acupressure

~ therapeutic massage

~ yoga or Tai Chi

8. Talk with your doctor or nurse about getting a referral to physical and occupational therapy for an exercise program and assistive devices to make activities of daily living easier.

Memory Changes (Cognitive Function)

Chemotherapy can injure the central nervous system (CNS), the part of the brain that coordinates muscle movement, reflexes, and thinking. Although women who have received chemotherapy have reported subtle changes in cognitive function or memory loss, these symptoms have in the past been overlooked. But that is true no longer. Among patients in support groups and networking classes, this memory change from chemotherapy is affectionately referred to as "chemobrain." Changes in memory, concentration, and language skills can occur up to two years after chemotherapy has been completed. These changes can be distressing for the individual, who may think she has something seriously wrong with her, such as a brain tumor or Alzheimer's disease. The patient should report any such symptoms to her doctor, who will want to determine the cause.

Besides chemotherapy, many other factors can affect concentration and memory: stress, anxiety, depression, and other medications. There are, however, specific chemotherapy agents that place the individual at increased risk for central nervous system toxicity. Toxicity generally occurs while the individual is receiving chemotherapy. The patient should report any of the following symptoms immediately to her doctor or nurse: blurred vision, slurred speech, difficulty walking, confusion, and seizures. The chemotherapy agent most often associated with CNS toxicity is ifosfamide; 5-FU also sometimes causes CNS toxicity, but less often. Chemotherapy with the offending agents will be discontinued if these side effects occur.

Patient Education for "Chemobrain"

1. Inform your doctor or nurse of any memory changes or muscle weakness.
2. Keep a "To Do" list to help plan and organize your activities.
3. Write down questions you have for your doctor or nurse, and bring the list with you to your appointment.
4. Bring a tape recorder to appointments if you have trouble remembering what has been said.
5. Reduce the stress in your life that you can control.
6. Play word games such as crossword puzzles or Scrabble to keep your brain exercising.

Hand-Foot Syndrome (Palmer-Planter Erythrodysesthesia)

Hand-foot syndrome (known as *Palmer-Planter Erythrodysesthesia*) is a condition in which the palms of the hands and the soles of the feet become red and dry, peel, and form blisters. Patients describe the skin sensations as anything from burning, with or without swelling, to severe pain. The cause is poorly understood. Several chemotherapy agents increase the risk of this side effect. The agents most commonly associated with hand-foot syndrome are 5-FU (5-fluorouracil), Doxil (liposomal doxorubicin), and Xeloda (capecitabine) (see Table 4.13). Although hand-foot symptoms are not life-threatening, they may interfere with daily activities, and chemotherapy may be delayed or stopped if the reaction is severe.

Hand-foot syndrome may appear after the first cycle of chemotherapy. Patients may not report it until it becomes severe or uncomfortable, but because it persists with each cycle of chemotherapy, patients are advised to inform their doctor or nurse of the earliest symptoms, such as redness or tingling of hands or feet. It's a good idea to avoid direct sunlight for the first three days after receiving Doxil or Xeloda, and to wear loose clothing, including shoes and socks that are not too tight and that do not cause pressure. Some patients have found that taking vitamin B_6 (pyridoxine) at a dose of 100 mg two to three times a day helps reduce or prevent hand-foot syndrome. Other soothing remedies are lanolin-based creams and lotions. Bag Balm is a petroleum-jelly-like lotion that is recommended for the feet; cover the feet with socks after applying Bag Balm. Your doc-

Table 4.13. Chemotherapy Used in Ovarian Cancer That Increases the Risk for Hand-Foot Syndrome

5-FU (5-fluorouracil)
Doxil (liposomal doxorubicin)
Xeloda (capecitabine)

tor may prescribe an anesthetic cream called Emla to soothe the burning feeling.

Patient Education for Hand-Foot Syndrome

1. Inform your doctor or nurse of any symptoms of hand-foot syndrome. These include redness of the skin, tingling, burning, swelling, or pain or tenderness on the palms of your hands or the soles of your feet.
2. Use lanolin-based creams and lotions on your feet and hands.
3. Ask your doctor or nurse about taking 100 mg of vitamin B_6 two to three times a day to prevent or reduce the severity of hand-foot syndrome.
4. Avoid direct sunlight for three days after receiving any chemotherapy known to cause hand-foot syndrome. Use sunscreen (SPF 15 or higher) at all times when you are out in the sunlight.
5. Avoid tight-fitting clothes, restrictive undergarments, and tight elastic waist or wrist bands.
6. Wear shoes and socks that are properly fitted and that do not cause pressure, rubbing, or blisters.
7. Avoid putting pressure on bony areas of your body (avoid kneeling and leaning on your elbows).

Conclusion

A woman's journey with ovarian cancer is personal and is unique to her. While many women have similar responses to the same treatment, nothing is more important than the individual's own experience and response.

In this chapter we have described certain specific side effects of chemotherapy. Other effects and reactions may occur also, depending on individual differences in height, weight, and prior medical history. The primary focus of this chapter has been to cover the more common ailments, to educate the patient and make her aware of potential problems so that intervention (and indeed prevention) can be instituted early, before the side effects become severe. Going through chemotherapy is not pleasant or easy. However, improvements continue to be made in managing the side effects of treatment that in years past would have caused women to stop treatment prematurely. Recognizing what to expect, when to call your doctor, and how to manage problems when they arise are all important components of your overall treatment program.

The health care team and the patient need to be partners in the patient's planned care and need to recognize and manage side effects early. Managing the side effects allows effective treatment to be given without interruption or delay, and it increases the potential for maintaining the patient's quality of life while she is having treatment. Collaboration between the patient and the health care team is the most effective strategy for the management of chemotherapy side effects and for achieving desirable physical and emotional outcomes, and thus for easing a woman's cancer journey.

Chapter 5

Radiation Therapy

This is a relatively short chapter, because radiation therapy has only a small and very restricted role in the management of ovarian cancer. In this chapter we look at the few instances in which radiation therapy is used in treating women with ovarian cancer.

Radiation therapy is a part of standard first-line therapy for many malignancies; for example, it provides an effective treatment for some women with cervical and endometrial cancer. It is not commonly used in the management of ovarian cancer, however—but not because it lacks effectiveness. On the contrary: ovarian cancer cells are relatively easily damaged and even killed by radiation therapy. Unfortunately, so are the normal cells surrounding the ovarian cancer cells. This problem often leads to toxicity or side effects that are intolerable and likely to harm the patient more than the radiation therapy is likely to help her.

Another reason for using radiation therapy only rarely to treat ovarian cancer is that ovarian cancer is not usually a localized disease. Because of this, a large area of the body would need to be radiated to be sure to include all areas where ovarian cancer cells may be found—so large that the cumulative toxicity of radiation therapy would lead to the patient's death. In short, the body just can't tolerate the radiation therapy needed to kill the ovarian cancer.

From the 1960s until the mid-1980s, some doctors recommended whole-abdominal radiation therapy to treat women who had multifocal residual disease noted at the time of a second-look procedure or following surgery for recurrent cancer. As mentioned above, the problem with this approach was not that the treatment did not successfully kill the remaining cancer in the area that was treated; the problem was that about 40 percent of the patients receiving this treatment suffered either disabling or fatal toxicity from the treatment. The disabling toxicity led to bowel obstructions, bowel impairments, and dependence on intravenous feedings. And, sadly, the patients' disease would recur anyway, in a part of the body away from the area that was radiated. This situation led to a general abandonment of whole-abdomen radiation therapy in the treatment of women with ovarian cancer except in very select circumstances.

Regardless of these realities, radiation therapy has been used in certain settings to treat ovarian cancer, and there are situations in which consideration may be given to using ionizing radiation as treatment. These four situations are described in the rest of this chapter.

Isolated Recurrence Treated with Full-Dose Radiation

We often consider and recommend radiation therapy for patients who

~ have undergone standard therapy,
~ have had a relatively long disease-free interval,
~ have an isolated recurrence (most commonly in a group of lymph nodes or in part of the pelvis),
~ have had the recurrence removed completely, and
~ to the best of our medical knowledge have no disease elsewhere (usually documented by extensive surgical restaging with numerous biopsies).

For a patient who meets all of these criteria, the side effects associated with administering full-dose external radiation therapy (about 50 Gray, the unit of measure most commonly employed) are limited and manageable, and the probability that the radiation therapy will kill any residual microscopic cells is high.

Intraperitoneal Radioactive Colloids for Early Isolated Disease with Positive Washings

There are numerous ways to administer radiation energy. One way is to use what are called *radioactive colloids*. These are particles in liquid form that can be placed in a cavity (such as the inside of the abdomen), where they deliver a dose of radiation therapy that can kill cancer cells over a short distance in any structure that the particles touch. The use of these materials was proposed for women with isolated disease in the ovary or ovaries when, even though the disease had been completely removed, washings in the abdomen had demonstrated the presence of cancer cells (called *FIGO Stage IC*; see Table 2.1 in Chapter 2).

The scientific rationale behind this method of treatment (referred to as *intraperitoneal radiation therapy*, or *IP radiation therapy*) made sense, and for a while this approach achieved a certain amount of popularity with doctors. The reality, however, is that, following surgery, adhesions form inside the abdomen that limit the distribution of the radioactive colloid. This means that not all surfaces get covered, and therefore larger areas of the peritoneal space become "sanctuaries" where cancer cells can literally hide from the intraperitoneal radiation therapy.

Unlike intraperitoneal chemotherapy, where the chemotherapeutic agent is absorbed into the bloodstream so that circulating tumor-killing doses occur, intraperitoneal radioactive colloids are only effective where they come in close proximity to the cancer cells. The sanctuaries that are created lead to disease recurrence. An additional disadvantage of the use of IP radioactive colloids is the risk that more adhesions (scar tissue) will form, blocking the intraperitoneal space. Such adhesions can increase the chances of a bowel obstruction developing as well as the likelihood of complications if any subsequent surgery is required. Given these limitations, IP radioactive colloid therapy is rarely used today, although it may be an option for some patients who cannot receive more standard methods of treatment, such as chemotherapy.

Germ Cell Neoplasms

Some malignancies arise from the germ cells (the cells that produce the eggs that eventually can be fertilized and lead to the development of an embryo). These malignancies, and particularly the ones called *dysgerminomas,* are exquisitely sensitive to radiation therapy. When these lesions have been surgically removed, and when it is known that the cancer has spread to local lymph nodes, radiation therapy to only that area is a rational choice.

Local radiation therapy is still used to treat dysgerminomas when chemotherapy has failed, when the patient chooses not to use chemotherapy, when the patient's medical condition precludes the use of chemotherapy, or because of other considerations. However, this treatment has fallen out of favor due to its side effects and because multi-agent chemotherapy has been demonstrated to be equally effective in treating dysgerminomas.

Whole-Abdominal Radiation

As mentioned earlier, whole-abdominal radiation therapy has largely been abandoned as a treatment for ovarian cancer because of the risk of associated complications. Nevertheless, it may still be considered as a treatment option in selected, extremely rare situations. Specifically, for patients with small-volume (less than a few millimeters) intraperitoneal disease in multiple sites who are unable or unwilling to take the more standard chemotherapy treatments, whole-abdominal radiation therapy may be offered, albeit with the risk of potentially disabling side effects.

As we said, this is a short chapter. Surgery and chemotherapy rather than radiation therapy are the mainstays of ovarian cancer treatment. When a doctor recommends radiation therapy for treating ovarian cancer, it is almost always in one of these select situations. The important point to appreciate is that every treatment decision involves a balance between potential benefit and potential risk, and radiation therapy is no different. Radiation therapy may be the best treatment for certain patients in selected situations, but the decision should only be made after careful consultation with your treating doctor.

Chapter 6

Nutrition

Western medicine, and specifically Western medicine as practiced in the United States, tends to assign nutrition a secondary role in the management of malignancies. We firmly believe
this approach is misguided at best and can be harmful to patients. It makes sense intuitively to consider adequate nutrition
as an essential part of treatment along with optimal surgery and
chemotherapy, and there is a growing catalog of scientific data
supporting this approach. Nutrition, for many health care pro-
fessions, has long been considered "complementary" therapy, but
because proper nutrition improves the outcome of treatment, we
treat our patients with nutrition as aggressively as we treat them
with surgery and chemotherapy.

   This chapter describes how ovarian cancer affects nutrition
and how nutritional support can improve the outcome of treatment for ovarian cancer. It also offers suggestions for maintaining a healthy diet during and after treatment.

How Does Ovarian Cancer Affect Nutrition?

Why are women with ovarian cancer malnourished in the first
place? There are three basic reasons, and for many women, all
three of these reasons come into play.

   First, a woman may have been malnourished before she developed ovarian cancer. Many Americans are amazed that they
can be "malnourished" while weighing more than they should!

Although this is not a unique phenomenon in the United States, it is something that we Americans seem to be better at than anyone else in the world. Left to their own devices, many people eat the wrong things, and too much of them. People who are obese are more likely than not to be malnourished: they have deficiencies in protein and other essential nutrients and vitamins as a result of their high-fat, high-complex-carbohydrate diets. The lean American is more likely to be nutritionally fit and often is more fit from a cardiovascular standpoint as well. But elderly people (and women with ovarian cancer commonly are elderly), particularly if they are poor or have limited financial resources, may be malnourished not only in proteins and other essential nutrients but also in total calorie intake.

Second, a woman may be malnourished because of the ovarian cancer itself. When ovarian cancer spreads outside of the ovaries, it often grows on the surface of the intestines and stomach or pushes on these structures. This growth can lead to narrowing and irritation of the intestines and stomach and can interfere with the woman's ability to take in or tolerate oral feedings, making it impossible for her to consume adequate calories and obtain necessary nutrients.

Finally, even a woman who is eating normally and healthily may become malnourished because the ovarian cancer consumes large amounts of calories and nutrients. Anything that is growing (like Rick's ten-year-old son, Jake) or that is metabolically very active (like his long-distance-running adult son, Rob) burns more calories than something that is not growing or not active. Ovarian cancer is both growing and very biologically active. Therefore, simply having ovarian cancer is a nutritional drain on the body.

How Does Nutrition Affect Treatment for Ovarian Cancer?

We have established why nutritional deficiencies are common in women with ovarian cancer. Now, what is the "cost" to the patient of these deficiencies?

Nutrition and Major Surgery

For centuries, surgeons have realized that malnourished patients are more likely to have complications following major surgery and are less likely to survive the operation. Malnutrition affects recovery from surgery in two basic ways: (1) impaired healing of the surgical site, whether the site of a bowel anastomosis (reconnection) or a site on the anterior (front) abdominal wall, and (2) the ability to resist and fight infection.

Wound Healing. For a surgical site to heal quickly and securely, the body must contain adequate amounts of essential protein, vitamins, and trace elements at the time of surgery. Many women with ovarian cancer, particularly if there has been a delay in the diagnosis and treatment of the malignancy, will have had some degree of intestinal dysfunction, as discussed earlier, causing a decrease in the intake of necessary nutrition. There may also be underlying issues of malnutrition associated with existing but unrelated medical problems such as diabetes, obesity (remember that many obese women are actually protein deficient), irritable or inflammatory bowel disease, and so on. Inadequate nutrition often leads to an increased possibility of wound separation, hernias, failure of intestinal anastomosis, and other problems.

Resisting and Fighting Infection. The human body cannot resist and fight infection as well when it has nutritional deficiencies as it does when it is well nourished. Because women who are having major surgical debulking procedures for ovarian cancer are undergoing a surgery that, although "clean," is commonly "contaminated" with bacteria, any failure in the body's ability to fight infections can be disastrous.

It's easy to see that the nutritional situation at the time of making the abdominal wall incision is extremely important. To improve a patient's nutritional well-being and increase the probability of a successful surgical outcome, it is recommended that a short period (about ten days) of intense nutritional supplementation be administered through intravenous feeding, either *total parenteral nutrition (TPN)* or *partial parenteral nutrition (PPN)*. *Parenteral* refers to the fact that the nutritional supplementation is bypassing the intestinal (enteral) tract (see below). We often delay surgery or chemotherapy to improve nutrition in women who are markedly nutritionally impaired.

Immune Function during Chemotherapy

The immune function is the body's mechanism to identify anything that is "different" or "foreign" and to kill it and clear it from the body. Maximal immune function is imperative for maximal cancer cell destruction. Because most chemotherapeutic regimens used to treat ovarian cancer lead to a decrease in the number of white blood cells (the cells that fight infection), it is essential for the white cells that *are* circulating to work as well as they can. Patients who are nutritionally impaired are more likely to have white cells that don't work as well at finding things that need to be killed and at killing them and clearing them from the body. In someone who is malnourished and undergoing chemotherapy, an impaired immune system can lead to less effective chemotherapy as well as an increased risk of infection and reduced ability to fight infection.

Achieving and Preserving Adequate Nutrition

As noted at the beginning of this chapter, we are as aggressive in nutritionally treating women with ovarian cancer as we are with our use of surgery and chemotherapy. For women with documented major nutritional abnormalities who are not able to consistently take in adequate oral nutrition (as shown by formal assessment during their hospitalization), we provide parenteral nutritional support until they have nutritionally "healed" and have demonstrated that they can receive adequate oral nutrition on a consistent basis. For many women, nutritional treatment is required for many weeks if not months, as the patient's nutritional deficit is corrected and the tumor load is decreased.

For a woman who does not have a nutritional deficiency at the time of diagnosis and initiation of therapy for ovarian cancer, everything that is possible must done to try to make sure that she remains nutritionally intact during her subsequent chemotherapy, for the reasons listed above. Chemotherapy has numerous side effects, and the management of these side effects is complex.

It is often difficult for a woman undergoing multi-agent chemotherapy to maintain adequate caloric and nutritional intake. This difficulty can be the result of gastrointestinal toxicity from the chemotherapy, appetite suppression from medications, and depression associated with the diagnosis of ovarian cancer, among other causes. Regardless of the cause or causes, a proactive approach must be taken to ensure that she does not develop a nutritional abnormality.

So far in this chapter we have discussed the very important topic of nutrition in women with ovarian cancer: how nutrition can be adversely affected by ovarian cancer and its treatment and why it is so important to maintain good nutrition. In the rest of the chapter we provide more specific information about nutritional needs and sources of nutrition that can be used as a woman is returning (it is hoped) to her pre-ovarian-cancer state.

Nutrition during Chemotherapy

For most women, eating a well-balanced diet that includes plenty of fruits, vegetables, and whole-grain products as well as a moderate amount of protein (low-fat meat) and dairy products is usually not difficult. For the reasons discussed earlier, however, ovarian cancer treatment and the side effects of treatment can compromise a woman's ability to consume a healthy diet. The specific side effects of treatment vary, depending on the chemotherapy drugs that are administered, although certain side effects are experienced by almost everyone to some degree.

The most common side effects of ovarian cancer chemotherapy treatment that may affect a woman's nutritional status are nausea, vomiting, loss of appetite, and a change in the sense of taste or smell. Diarrhea and constipation may also occur, although they are less common. Chemotherapy can lead to a general sense of fatigue, sometimes meaning you are just too tired to prepare and eat a proper meal. Rarely, chemotherapy treatments can cause sores to form in the mouth and throat and make it physically painful to swallow food or liquid; this situation can lead to malnutrition and dehydration.

Although these side effects are time limited (they will go away after treatment is completed), they can make it very difficult to maintain your strength during therapy. To help maintain your strength during chemotherapy, we suggest you follow some or all of the following suggestions.

Maintain a Positive Attitude. Maintaining a positive attitude is critical to the process of surviving ovarian cancer. Take a positive attitude about improving your overall health and your body's ability to get through treatment by attending to your nutritional needs and maintaining your strength. Be proactive about deciding what you put in your body. Focus on seeing nutrition, along with exercise and getting plenty of sleep, as an important part of a healthy lifestyle, which is conducive to maintaining a positive attitude.

Develop a Nutritional Plan. Before beginning chemotherapy treatment, we always recommend that our patients have a formal consultation with an experienced dietician or nutritionist to develop an individual nutritional plan or program. These professionals are familiar with how cancer treatment can affect nutritional intake and will design a dietary regimen based on your personal likes and dislikes that still satisfies your nutritional needs. Eating is much easier if you are eating foods that you like, even if it means eating for dinner what you would normally eat for breakfast.

It is important to include foods with high caloric and nutritional value, especially those that contain potassium, calcium, iron, and magnesium, as these foods will help your body recover from surgery and alleviate some of the side effects of chemotherapy. Supplementing meals with nutritious snacks can be a good source of extra calories and protein (see Table 6.1). Try to keep a variety of snacks on hand that you can eat during the day and that are easy to prepare. Suggestions include soup, cereal and milk, yogurt, and half a sandwich. Be careful to avoid snacks that might make the side effects of chemotherapy treatment worse (for example, don't eat large amounts of fruits and raw vegetables if you are having diarrhea). Our patients have found it very helpful to meet with their dietician periodically throughout the course of treatment, to review how their nutritional program is working for them and make any necessary adjustments.

Plan Ahead. After you have developed your nutritional plan, spend some time thinking about what foods you will need a week or two in advance. Stock up on food products while you are feeling well enough to go shopping (don't wait until right after a treatment when fatigue will be the most noticeable). It is also a good idea to prepare some of your meals in advance, so you won't have to do as much cooking immediately after each treatment.

Make Use of All Your Resources. Don't be afraid to ask your family and friends to help you with your nutritional program. They can shop for you and prepare foods and meals. Family and friends are usually anxious and willing to participate in your care. Helping with shopping and cooking is a great way to get them directly involved and give them the satisfaction of knowing that they are actively helping you to get better and stronger.

Make Sure You Are Obtaining the Necessary Nutrients. Side effects of treatment, such as persistent nausea or mouth sores, can prevent you from consuming adequate calories. In addition, ovarian cancer itself can cause problems, such as a partial bowel obstruction, that make it difficult to stay adequately nourished. Although not ideal, there are several alternatives to eating by mouth in these circumstances.

A *gastric feeding tube* is a thin, flexible tube that is placed directly into the stomach through the abdominal wall. Once in

Table 6.1. Examples of Nutritious Snacks

Angel food cake	Fruit—fresh, canned, dried	Peanut butter
Bread		Popcorn, pretzels
Cereal—hot or cold	Gelatin	Puddings, custards
Cheese	Granola	Sandwiches
Cookies	Homemade milk-shakes and drinks	Sherbet
Crackers	Ice cream	Soups—broth based or hearty
Dips made with cheese, beans, and yogurt	Juices	Sports drinks
	Milk	Vegetables—raw, cooked
Eggnog (pasteurized)	Muffins	
	Nuts	Yogurt—carton, frozen

place, high-calorie nutrition formulas can be delivered through the tube. Feeding tubes are used when someone is unable to physically eat but still has a functioning intestinal (digestive) tract. Ideally, oral intake should be resumed as soon as possible.

Parenteral nutrition can be used when there is a serious problem with the digestive tract, such as partial obstruction, severe vomiting, or diarrhea, and adequate nutrients cannot be absorbed from the intestines. Parenteral nutrition involves administering a nutritional solution through the vein (intravenously). Both gastric tube and parenteral nutrition can be given at home.

After Treatment Ends

Most of the side effects of chemotherapy will dissipate within a few weeks of completing the final treatment. If problems such as poor appetite or a change in taste or smell persist longer than this, it is a good idea to talk with your doctor, nurse, or dietician to develop a plan to address the issue. Eating well and maintaining good nutritional status after your treatment has ended is an excellent way to regain your strength, rebuild tissue, improve your energy level, and feel better overall.

Chapter 7

Controlling Pain and Suffering

Pain and suffering are two very different processes, although many people, including health care professionals, often (inaccurately) equate the two. In this chapter we discuss these two different but related processes separately, just as we believe they need to be managed separately.

Dealing with Pain

In the 1980s the experts at the Memorial Sloan-Kettering Cancer Institute in New York City championed the development of an objective measure of pain, which they called the Fifth Vital Sign. (The other four vital signs are temperature; heart rate; breathing, or respiration, rate; and blood pressure.) The formalization of pain as a vital sign was a great incentive to develop a *linear analogue scale measure of pain,* a well-validated and easy-to-reproduce way of measuring a patient's discomfort. The pain scale that is used at the Johns Hopkins Hospital and Medical Institutions is shown on the next page.

Whenever a patient is receiving medications or other therapy for pain or is experiencing pain, the health care provider needs to measure the patient's pain often and objectively, using the pain scale instrument. We do this as part of our routine with every visit that a patient makes to our consultation suite, and we store the data as part of our patient's medical record. This allows

(For Addressograph Plate)

PATIENT INSTRUCTIONS: This questionnaire helps the physicians and nurses evaluate your health and plan your care. Please answer all questions using a <u>PEN</u>.

ADULT PATIENT: Circle the number from 0-10 that best describes how much pain you are having **right now.**

```
0   1   2   3   4   5   6   7   8   9   10
|---|---|---|---|---|---|---|---|---|---|
```

No Pain   Worst Possible Pain

Numerical Pain Rating Scale

FOR A CHILD (3 years old +) OR NON-ENGLISH SPEAKING ADULT · Circle the face that best describes how you feel **right now.**

0	1	2	3	4	5
No Hurt	Hurts Little Bit	Hurts Little More	Hurts Even More	Hurts Whole Lot	Hurts Worst

Wong-Baker Faces Pain Rating Scale, from Wong, D.L., Hockenberry-Eaton, M., Wilson, D., Winkelstein, M.L., Schwartz, P.: Wong's Essentials of ediatric Nursing, ed. 6, St. Louis, 2001, p. 1301. Copyrighted by Mosby, Inc. Reprinted by permission.

DO YOU WANT YOUR DOCTOR TO ADDRESS YOUR PAIN DURING TODAY'S VISIT?   ☐ Yes   ☐ No

LIST ANY MEDICATIONS OR TREATMENTS THAT YOU ARE USING FOR PAIN RELIEF:

_____

_____

_____

Patient Signature: _____   **Date:** _____

FOR PROVIDER USE ONLY:

Complete the following section of this form, if the patient has:
- a **pain rating > 3** on the **numerical** pain rating scale, **or,**
- a **pain rating > 1** on the **Faces** scale, **or,**
- indicated the desire to have his/her pain addressed during today's visit.

Check appropriate box below:

        ☐ **Pain assessed and managed**
        ☐ **Pain assessed and patient advised about/referred for pain management**
        ☐ **Patient referred for assessment and pain management**

Provider signature: _____   **ID:** _____   **Date:** _____

us to routinely reassess how severe a patient's pain is and whether there has been improvement.

It is commonly said that simply admitting a problem exists is the most important step in solving it. Sadly, that's not always true. Although we now have a great way to measure pain, we health care professionals are, in general, deficient in making sure that our patients have adequate pain control. We are not solely to blame for this problem, though. Even when health care professionals are able to provide adequate pain relief, some patients have difficulty with or refuse to comply with our pain control recommendations.

Why don't patients have adequate pain control? Not surprisingly, there are numerous reasons. Some of these barriers to adequate pain control are legitimate, but the majority are not. In this list, we consider only the first two to be legitimate.

1. Patients' intolerance of side effects of pain medications.
2. Patients' inability to afford pain medications.
3. Health care professionals' ignorance about how to control complex and severe pain.
4. Health care professionals' unwillingness to administer adequate drugs because of fear that the patient will become addicted.
5. Patients' unwillingness to take adequate drugs because of fear of becoming addicted.
6. Patients' inability to understand or comply with the complexity of a pain treatment regimen.

Patients Who Have Trouble Tolerating Side Effects

Side effects of pain medication are a real problem for patients, particularly when the patient is just being started on relatively high doses of medications. We have two ways to improve patient tolerance. First, we try to do a stepwise increase in the drugs that are being administered. This means not only changing drug doses one at a time and in a graduated fashion but also adding new drugs and different drugs one at a time and avoiding simultaneously adding new drugs and increasing doses.

Second, we anticipate side effects, informing the patient that the side effect may occur and preemptively treating the side effect or administering something that can minimize the side effect. Having ovarian cancer forces patients to lose control over their lives. Not knowing what sort of side effects can occur and then to have something unpleasant happen is another instance of "control loss"—a situation we actively try to avoid for our patients. There is so little that an ovarian cancer patient can control that whenever we can return control of anything to one of our patients, we will do so.

A classic example of a side effect related to narcotic administration that can be anticipated and minimized is constipation. Every patient taking any type of "real" pain medications (from Tylenol #3 or Tylox to MS-Contin or Oxycontin) will have some degree of constipation. We start all of our patients who are taking narcotic medications on stool softeners and bulking agents, and we review with them the need to make sure they are drinking plenty of noncaffeinated liquids (eight, eight-ounce glasses each day at a minimum) as well as bulky foods (whole grains, fresh fruits and veggies, and so on), while avoiding constipating foods such as those in the BRAT diet (bananas, rice, applesauce, and toast) or anything "white" (such as white bread, white rice, and white potatoes).

Patients Who Cannot Afford Pain Medications

Unfortunately, this is not an uncommon reality for ovarian cancer patients and other patients with malignancies. According to the U.S. Department of Health and Human Services, in the spring of 2002 there were approximately 41 million Americans who did not have insurance coverage. These fellow citizens, of course, are lacking prescription benefits. Furthermore, even many individuals who do have insurance do not have prescription benefits.

Medicare is a common primary insurer for American women with ovarian cancer. As the reader probably appreciates, although there have been attempts to enact a prescription benefit package for Medicare recipients, an ideal solution does not yet exist. Recognizing that many people live on a limited income, and considering the high cost of one drug prescription—let alone several prescriptions—it is evident that the cost of prescriptions for someone with ovarian cancer can be a big hit on a limited budget. Fortunately, many of the pharmaceutical companies have programs for supplying subsidized medications. But a great deal of paperwork must be done to obtain these benefits. As a group of health care professionals committed to eliminating suffering wherever possible, we feel the time has come to have a comprehensive prescription benefit for Medicare patients.

Health Care Professionals Who Don't Know How to Control Complex and Severe Pain

Pain associated with recurrent malignancies can be some of the most difficult pain to manage. There are malignancies both of the female genital tract (cervix) and elsewhere (lung and breast) that can present a difficult challenge for the doctor and the patient in achieving adequate analgesia. Fortunately for most women who have ovarian cancer, the pain associated with the treatment (most commonly surgical) of the disease can be relatively easily controlled using straightforward and generally well-tolerated drugs and other methods. And most women who have recurrent or even end-of-life ovarian cancer do not have pain that is difficult to control.

The optimal management of any but the lowest level of pain is outlined in the "Triad of Treatment":

1. Narcotics
    ~ Short-acting
    ~ Long-acting
2. Anti-inflammatories
3. Potentiators
    ~ Neuroleptics
    ~ Antidepressants

~ Anti-anxiety agents
~ Others

Narcotics. Although narcotics are the leading edge of the triad, their use is not well understood by the lay person and even by some clinicians. On the one hand, narcotic medications can be very fast-acting and last only a short time (such as the elixir and intravenous formats), having "half-lives" (how long a meaningful circulating level of the drug is in the bloodstream) of only a few minutes. On the other hand, some narcotic medications take hours or days to reach their maximal effect and have a long-lasting half-life (of twelve to fifteen hours) or a continuous effect (such as that achieved through transdermal delivery systems). (See Table 7.1.)

There are some general rules that we like to follow when prescribing narcotic pain medications that the layperson should be aware of:

First, we start with a narcotic pain medication that lasts about four to six hours. If a person needs to take her pain medication more frequently than that, she should either receive a higher dose of the intermediate-acting medication or be started on a longer-acting medication.

Second, if we anticipate that the pain will be getting better quickly and will last a relatively short time (like the pain that accompanies a major surgical procedure), we will use the intermediate-half-life narcotic medications. However, if the pain is not resolving after a few weeks and the patient needs to take many pills at a time just to get adequate relief, we will quickly add a more potent or a longer-lasting narcotic medication.

Finally, severe or "aggressive" pain needs aggressive treatment. Although it is important to increase narcotic medications in an appropriate stepwise fashion (adding about 30 percent of relative analgesic effect with each change), these changes can be made frequently (every seventy-two hours, more or less, depending upon which medication is used).

Table 7.1. Half-Lives and Side Effects of Common Narcotic
Pain Medications

Medication	Half-Life (hours)	Side Effects
Codeine	2–3	Drowsiness, dizziness, confusion, constipation
Oxycodone	2–3	Drowsiness, dizziness, confusion, constipation, nausea and vomiting
Morphine	2–3	Drowsiness, dizziness, confusion, headache, constipation, nausea and vomiting, itching
Hydromorphone	2–3	Drowsiness, confusion, headache, flushing, low blood pressure, palpitations, nausea and vomiting, stomach cramps
Levorphanol	12–15	Drowsiness, confusion, headache, flushing, low blood pressure, palpitations, itching, nausea and vomiting, stomach cramps
Fentanyl (transdermal)*		Drowsiness, confusion, low blood pressure, slow heart rate, nausea and vomiting, constipation

*Transdermal delivery systems have duration of action lasting from 48
to 72 hours.

Anti-Inflammatories. Anti-inflammatory medications, also called
nonsteroidal anti-inflammatory drugs, or NSAIDs (see Table 7.2),
are valuable additions to narcotic pain medications and can also
be substituted for narcotic pain medications. We start almost all
of our postoperative patients on a long-acting, nonsteroidal anti-
inflammatory agent as soon as they are taking any meaningful
amount of liquids or solids orally. The early use of NSAIDs has

Table 7.2. Half-Lives and Side Effects of Common NSAID
Pain Medications

Medication	Half-Life (hours)	Side Effects
Aspirin	3–12	Bleeding, low blood pressure, confusion, nausea, heartburn, stomach ulcers, rash
Acetaminophen	3–4	Low blood counts, kidney damage
Ibuprofen	3–4	Headache, fatigue, itching, rash, vomiting, stomach ulcers, heartburn, diarrhea, constipation
Indomethacin	4–5	Headache, dizziness, nausea, constipation, stomach cramps, bleeding
Ketorolac	4–7	Edema, headache, dizziness, stomach pain, diarrhea, rash

been repeatedly demonstrated to decrease the total amount of
narcotic pain medication necessary to obtain adequate pain control, therefore decreasing many of the unpleasant side effects of
narcotic pain medication.

Similarly, as soon as it becomes clear that a patient is going
to require long-term pain medications, we will add NSAIDs to
the pain-medication regimen, whether or not she is in the postoperative period. *Steroidal* anti-inflammatory medications are
not used as part of pain control, simply because of the side effects (toxicity) of these medications. The risk-benefit ratio, except in certain unique acute settings, is just too high.

Potentiators. The potentiators include a wide variety of drugs,
many of which act by preventing the transmission of pain signals
by the nerves. Others may have a more central action, serving as
an antidepressant or anxiolytic (anti-anxiety medication) (see
Table 7.3). Every expert has a preference among the potentiator
drugs, but selecting a medication depends in great part upon the

Table 7.3. Side Effects of Common Potentiator Pain
Medications

Medication	Side Effects
Antidepressants	
Amitriptyline	Restlessness, dizziness, insomnia, rash, weight gain, constipation
Paroxetine	Headache, dizziness, nausea, constipation, diarrhea, low blood pressure
Venlafaxine	Headache, dizziness, somnolence, insomnia, nausea, constipation, anorexia, weakness, rash
Neuroleptics	
Gabapentin	Drowsiness, dizziness, fatigue, edema, nausea and vomiting, itching
Anti-anxiety agents	
Lorazepam	Sedation, low blood pressure, headache, nausea, rash, nasal congestion

type and location of the patient's pain and what other medications she may need. For this reason, the choice of potentiator
varies from patient to patient. In general, we will add a neu-
roleptic medication such as gabapentin and an anxiolytic agent
(such as lorazepam), or an antidepression agent (venlafaxine or
a similar drug), or a combination, to the regimen of short- and
long-acting narcotics and NSAIDs. Even though this may mean
that a patient is taking five different medications to control her
pain, the inconvenience of taking the meds is offset by the successful control of pain and the improvement in the patient's
quality of life.

Non-Oral Means of Delivering Medications. Another available
option is to use more invasive means of pain control for patients
who are unable to tolerate oral medications or for whom adequate pain relief just cannot be obtained. The choices that

patients have include simple systems such as a transdermal delivery system, which is a patch worn on the skin that is changed every few days and that delivers a continuous level of a narcotic. More complex regimens that are available involve the use of either intravenous (in a vein) or subcutaneous (under the skin) infusion systems or a catheter (such as epidural or intrathecal) so that analgesics can be infused around the nerves (intrathecally) to anesthetize the nerves and block the transmission of the pain sensation.

Health Care Professionals Who Are Concerned That the Patient Will Become Addicted

Any number of misunderstandings on the part of health care professionals can interfere with the delivery of optimal patient care. This is one of them. Addiction is both a physiological and a psychological process. Patients who need pain medications to control their discomfort and to allow them to live a life as close to normal as possible do not become "addicted" to the medications that are prescribed.

It's true that over time the patients may need a higher dose of pain medication as they become acclimated to the drugs they are receiving or when the disease progresses. Either of these situations may mean the patient requires more medication to control more pain. And of course, when medications that have been used for a long time in relatively high doses are stopped, there will be symptoms. Though these symptoms could theoretically be labeled as withdrawal, that is an overstatement. For example, Rick takes Lipitor to control his elevated cholesterol levels. If he stopped the Lipitor, his cholesterol would go back up and he would have some "withdrawal" symptoms (less constipation!). He is not addicted to Lipitor, but he uses it for the treatment of a disease process. The same is true of medications to treat cancer pain. *Pain associated with cancer is a disease that deserves treatment, and pain medications are the medically advised best treatment.*

Patients Who Are Afraid of Becoming Addicted

We discussed this issue indirectly above, in the section on health care professionals' concerns about patients' addiction. In our view, doctors and nurses really have an obligation to make sure that patients understand that they will not become addicted but will become healthier. It's worth repeating: Pain associated with cancer is a disease that deserves treatment, and pain medications are the medically advised best treatment. Take the pain medications that are recommended to you!

Many patients also may have a difficult time confessing to themselves that they are actually having significant amounts of pain. We believe that a lot of patients, though they won't acknowledge it, view the reality that they are having pain as an indication that their cancer is not controlled or is progressing. In some instances this is true, but in most instances it is not. Doctors and nurses must share with the ovarian cancer patient the information that some degree of pain is a normal part of the recovery from surgery and the associated treatment of cancer. Acknowledging the pain that one is having is not being weak, nor is it accepting "failure." It is being honest with oneself and one's care providers. Enough said.

Patients Who Cannot Understand or Comply with a Pain Treatment Regimen

The therapeutic regimens that we described earlier in this chapter can be complex, and it may be difficult for patients with limited intellectual capacity, compromised mental acuity as a result of age or disease, or limited dexterity to comply with the regimens. In the effort to make patients independent and as free from restrictions as possible, doctors generally prescribe oral medications, rather than placing patients on regimens that are given by a parenteral (non-oral) route, such as intravenous administration or intramuscular injections, or that require skilled nursing help to administer.

There are regimens that require fewer oral medications, such as those using a transdermal delivery system (the "patch") or infusion pumps. The problems with the patch are cost and local skin irritation, and the problems with infusion pumps are cost and the need for skilled assistance in placing the subcutaneous needle, changing the pump, and so on. We have found that with a simplified regimen that is explicitly outlined and printed out for the patient, the patient, or at least her care partner, is able to master the schedules for oral medications.

Dealing with Suffering

Physical pain, which can be quantified and explained on a physiological basis, can be a cause of suffering, but it is far from the only source of suffering for patients with ovarian cancer. Suffering is located much more on a spiritual or metaphysical plane. We personally believe that for most of our patients, suffering is more of an issue than pain is. But in contrast with pain control, there is no well-validated and scientifically proved algorithm for the management of suffering. We do, however, have an approach that over the years we have employed successfully in helping patients.

First, we broach the issue. That doesn't mean that we blurt out "Are you suffering?" It means that we will ask patients, in an open fashion, "How are you doing with your cancer?" or something similar. This issue is raised after we have asked our series of specific questions that we need specific answers to (regarding gastrointestinal and genitourinary function, function of arms and legs, cardiovascular and pulmonary function, vaginal and sexual function, and so on). When given the opportunity to express how they feel, most patients will open up to some degree. Though suffering cannot be cured simply by acknowledging that it is present, there is no doubt in our minds that such an acknowledgment helps.

We give the patient the right to suffer. This statement may seem remarkably paternalistic, and almost cruel, but again, we have found that for our patients it is often helpful to allow them the right to suffer. The majority of patients play the "tough role," acting stoic. There is, of course, value in playing that role, but it doesn't really allow a patient to come to peace with what is happening to her and to those around her. Simply acknowledging that her "heart" is hurting, that she is suffering, and that it is ok to feel that way will go a long way toward opening up avenues for decreasing the suffering.

We use professionals. We are not psychologists, social workers, group therapists, priests, rabbis, pastors, or members of any other group with professional training in relieving spiritual and psychic suffering. But we rely on a large group of professionals to whom we refer our patients. It is important to recognize that what works for one individual and her family may not work for the next. However, something works for everyone if enough effort is put forth to discover what that "something" is and to address the critical issues.

We ask again. We don't assume because a patient has been willing to open up to us and share with us that she is suffering and because we have given her the appropriate referral that the issue is resolved and is no longer "our problem." In contrast to that approach, every time we see a patient, we will ask the same questions, always offering some intervention.

We consider the use of psychoactive drugs. We don't follow the rule of Rick's grandfather, an old-time general doc who practiced in the middle half of the last century, that every patient we see needs to leave with some new medication that we give her. However, there are a significant number of patients who do have either a reactive depression or an anxiety as a result of their ovarian cancer diagnosis and the treatment or the natural course the disease has taken. For any patient who meets the diagnostic criteria of either depression or an anxiety disorder, we will institute first-line pharmacotherapy and provide a referral to a mental health care professional. We only write prescriptions for a small amount of medications (usually thirty to forty-five days' worth), and we repeatedly stress to our patients that we are instituting a therapy that we are comfortable with but that we want them to have long-term professional follow-up with a mental health expert.

It is important for the reader to hear again: we consider the management and preferably the elimination of suffering to be as important a goal as the curing of cancer. It is our opinion that there definitely are fates that are "worse than death." Emotional torment is one of them.

Chapter 8

Complementary and Alternative Medicine Therapies

National surveys have confirmed a continual increase in the use of complementary and alternative medicine (CAM) therapies in the United States and Europe. The term *alternative* used to be used as an umbrella term to describe the therapies not taught in U.S. medical schools or provided in U.S. hospitals. Now, because many medical schools currently include these therapies in their curricula, and some of the therapies are currently provided to patients in hospitals and cancer centers, the term is no longer appropriate or accurate.

The interchangeable use of the terms *complementary* and *alternative* has led to miscommunication and confusion among health care providers and the public and between patients and health care providers. These terms are not interchangeable. *Complementary* and *alternative* describe the intent with which a therapy is used, not the therapy itself. A therapy is "alternative" when it is used *instead of* conventional therapy. "Complementary" therapies are those used *in addition to,* or *to complement,* conventional therapy. We prefer the more contemporary term *integrative medicine,* which reflects the use of CAM therapies in combination with conventional therapies. In this framework, CAM therapies are used to reduce or ameliorate the side effects of conventional treatments (such as chemotherapy) or to strengthen the body, for example through enhanced nutrition, to help a person tolerate conventional cancer treatments.

We are learning more about CAM therapies, but there is still much to be discovered about the safety, efficacy, action, and potential adverse effects of these therapies. In a 1990 survey, 9 percent of five thousand persons with cancer reported using these therapies. Ten years later, a CAM therapy survey showed that patients with cancer who were participating in clinical trials used spirituality (94%); imagery (86%); massage (80%); lifestyle, diet, or nutrition (60%); relaxation (50%); herbal or botanical substances (20%); and high-dose vitamins (14%). Other surveys report that the use of CAM therapy by persons with cancer ranges from 50 to 83 percent.

It is vitally important for you to tell your doctor or nurse about any CAM therapies that you are using. Rather than being quick to discourage the use of all such therapies, your health care provider will want to make sure that a particular CAM therapy (herbal supplements, for example) is safe and will not compromise the effectiveness of any conventional treatment you may be receiving.

Before beginning any CAM therapy, you should consult with an experienced CAM practitioner. Your doctor or nurse can be a good source of information, and many cancer centers now include entire departments devoted to integrating CAM therapies with conventional cancer treatments. Persons with cancer (or well-meaning family and friends) will often seek assistance at their local health food store. It is important to remember that while the person working in a health food store may be knowledgeable about products, he or she does not have enough information or knowledge about the patient's diagnosis (or diagnoses) and all the medications involved to make a safe and appropriate recommendation. Also, some CAM practitioners promote themselves as having a cure for cancer. If it is a "cure" or a "secret cure," remember: *If it sounds too good to be true, it usually is.* There are no secrets.

The National Institutes of Health–National Center for Complementary and Alternative Medicine (NIH-NCCAM) was created in 1998 to evaluate alternative medical treatment modalities in order to determine their effectiveness. The NCCAM does not provide referrals for CAM therapies or practitioners. It does, however, support research and training and provide information on CAM therapies (see its Web site at www.nccam.nih.gov). This center describes seven categories and five domains of CAM therapies (see Table 8.1).

Not all CAM therapies are directly applicable to women with ovarian cancer. In the following sections we have summarized some of the therapies that our patients have found to be most helpful in relieving symptoms and improving the quality of life by reducing side effects of conventional treatments or by providing psychological benefits. We also present a brief summary of some of the more commonly encountered herbs and dietary supplements; however, we reiterate that these herbs and supplements should not be used as alternatives to conventional treatments to fight cancer.

Mind, Body, and Spirit Methods

Aromatherapy

Aromatherapy is the use of essential oils (fragrant substances distilled from plants) to alter mood or improve health. Essential oils are highly concentrated aromatic substances that can be either inhaled or applied as oils during therapeutic massage. For inhalation, steaming water, diffusers, or humidifiers are used to spread a combination of the steam and a few drops of the essential oil throughout the room. For skin application, essential oils are usually mixed with vegetable oil and massaged directly into the skin.

Aromatherapy can enhance the quality of life as a complementary treatment: it can reduce stress, pain, and depression and produce a feeling of well-being. There are more than forty different essential oils; the most commonly used are lavender, eucalyptus, rosemary, jasmine, chamomile, peppermint, and geranium. Lavender oil is promoted to reduce stress, anxiety, insomnia, and muscle tension. Inhaled peppermint and ginger oil

Table 8.1. A Brief Description of Complementary and Alternative Medicine Therapy Categories

Alternative Systems of Medical Care
These systems stress prevention of disease and promotion of health that includes personal responsibility. The alternative systems are a way of being and a way of living that promote balance in all aspects of one's life. Examples include Traditional Chinese Medicine (TCM), naturopathy, and homeopathy.

Mind-Body Medicine
Understanding that the body is influenced by the mind is not new. Mind-body medicine therapies are based on the connection of the mind to the body—and the potential for a person to influence his or her own healing. Examples include meditation, guided imagery or visualization, relaxation, and creative art therapies. Controversy exists over whether mind-body medicine improves quality of life or survival time. Those with a history of clinical depression, bipolar disorder, or schizophrenia should check with their mental health professional prior to using these therapies.

Bioelectromagnetic Therapies
The use of acupuncture is well researched, and it is recognized in pain management therapy. We are learning more about the use of acupuncture in other clinical conditions, as well. The contemporary use of magnets has stimulated discussion regarding the use of magnets for pain relief and health promotion.

Herbal Medicine
The goal of herbal medicine is to assist the body to restore and maintain balance. Herbal remedies can be taken internally or applied to the skin. Just because herbs are "natural" does not mean they are necessarily safe. Herbs have the ability to interact with each other and with pharmaceuticals (drugs) as well as with supplements. Herbs should be discontinued if any unpleasant side effects occur; when in doubt, do without.

Pharmacological and Biological Therapies
These therapies have what some have referred to as "the lure of the cure." They claim to cure everything from obesity to cancer.

(continued)

Table 8.1. *Continued*

Scientific proof may be lacking for many of these therapies. Examples include laetrile and shark cartilage.

Manual Healing Methods
Manual healing methods involve touch. These therapies appeal to us because human beings (in our culture) have a strong desire to touch and be touched. Examples include Reiki, chiropractic, reflexology, massage, therapeutic touch or healing touch (the last is a misnomer, since actual touch may not be involved). Caution should be taken with regard to massage for people with certain clinical conditions.

Diet, Nutrition, and Lifestyle Changes
Much has been written about nutrition and its effect on health and disease. Caution should be taken with very restrictive dietary programs. There are controversies regarding the effects of antioxidants and/or vitamins during certain cancer therapies. These controversies include the question of dietary soy (which is good for some kinds of cancer and controversial or risky for others). Examples of CAM diet therapies include macrobiotics, the Gerson program, and the Gonzalez regimen.

---

may help to reduce chemotherapy-related nausea, although the reports of this effect have not been scientifically proved.

Aromatherapy may be self-administered or practiced by an aromatherapist. Many aromatherapists are also trained as massage therapists, psychologists, chiropractors, or social workers. It may be advisable to seek a consultation from someone experienced in aromatherapy before starting treatment, particularly when applying essential oils directly to the skin. Essential oils should never be taken internally (many of them are poisonous if ingested) or applied for prolonged periods of time. There is no scientific evidence to support aromatherapy as a means of preventing or treating cancer.

Art Therapy

Art therapy uses creative activities to express emotions and provides a way for people to increase self-awareness, express unspoken concerns about their disease, or come to terms with emotional conflicts. A trained art therapist usually serves as a facilitator while patients work individually or in groups to express themselves through their art and discuss emotions and concerns as they relate to their creations. Many cancer centers and support groups are able to provide access to a trained art therapist.

Imagery

The complementary therapy of imagery uses visualization techniques and mental exercises to enable the mind to influence the health and well-being of the body. While imagery does not appear to directly affect cancer growth, the techniques of imagery can help reduce anxiety, improve depression, and create feelings of being in control, and thus they may be helpful in reducing pain. For cancer patients, imagery has been promoted as a way to alleviate the nausea caused by chemotherapy and reduce the stress associated with having cancer. Guided imagery is one technique that entails visualizing a specific goal to be achieved and imagining achieving that goal, much as an athlete would do before beginning a competition. Imagery techniques should be guided by a trained health care provider, at least at the start of therapy, and are best used as a complementary therapy to conventional treatments.

Meditation

Meditation is a relaxation method that can be useful as a complementary therapy for treating chronic pain and insomnia and improving the overall quality of life. There is no evidence that meditation is effective in directly treating cancer, however. There are different types of meditation that use concentration or reflection to relax the body and calm the mind to create a sense of well-being. Meditation can be self-directed or guided by a health care professional. In self-directed meditation, one sits or rests in a quiet place free from noise and distraction, trying to achieve a feeling of peace. A relaxed yet alert state is created by concentrating on a pleasant idea or thought, chanting a special phrase or sound, or focusing on the sound of one's breathing. A mental separation from the outside world is the goal of meditation, which is promoted as a way of reducing stress on both the mind and the body.

Tai Chi

Tai Chi is a mind-body self-healing system that is an ancient Chinese form of martial arts using movement, meditation, and breathing to improve health and well-being. Tai Chi is based on the theory of yin and yang (the interaction of opposite forces) and is thought to balance the flow of vital energy or life force (called *chi*) to improve general health and extend life. It incorporates slow, graceful movements with rhythmic breathing to relax the body as well as the mind and reduce stress. The deep breathing and physical movements are a good source of exercise and are associated with improved posture, flexibility, agility, balance, and circulation. Meditative concentration focuses on a point just below the navel, from which it is thought that *chi* radiates throughout the body, as a series of gentle, deliberate movements called forms are performed. Each form consists of twenty to one hundred individual movements and is named from nature (for example, "Wave hands like a cloud"). Tai Chi can be a useful adjunct to conventional therapy, especially as part of a physical rehabilitation program after surgery; however, there is no evidence that it can cure or prevent cancer.

Yoga

Yoga is a form of nonaerobic exercise based on a program of precise posture and breathing techniques. Yoga is thought to cultivate *prana,* which means vital energy or life force and is similar to *chi* in traditional Chinese medicine. As a way of life, yoga is based on Hindu traditions that combine physical exercise, meditation, dietary guidelines, and ethical standards to create a union of mind, body, and spirit. Similar to Tai Chi, yoga can provide a good source of exercise and serve to increase strength and reduce stress.

There are different variations of yoga; the more common types incorporate physical movement, breathing exercises, and meditation to achieve a connection between the mind, body, and spirit. A typical yoga session may include guided imagery or visualization, in addition to gentle movements and breathing, and may last from twenty minutes to an hour. Yoga can be practiced at home without an instructor, but beginners are urged to start with an educational class or classes at a yoga center, local community center, or health club. Although yoga can provide an improved level of fitness, reduce stress, and increase feelings of relaxation and well-being, there is no evidence that it is effective in treating or preventing cancer.

Manual Healing and Physical Touch Methods

Acupuncture

Acupuncture is a CAM therapy in which very thin needles are inserted through the skin at various locations called *acupoints*. In Chinese medicine, acupuncture is used as an anesthetic during surgery and to relieve the symptoms of a variety of conditions, and it is believed to have the power to cure certain diseases. It is thought that acupoints lie along invisible meridians, which are channels for the flow of vital energy of life force (called *chi*). Needles are inserted just beneath the skin at specific acupoints and are thought to restore balance and a healthy energy flow to the body. Skilled acupuncturists cause virtually no pain. Although there is no scientific evidence that acupuncture can cure cancer, an expert panel from the National Institutes of Health concluded that acupuncture is an effective treatment for nausea caused by chemotherapy drugs and may lessen the need for conventional pain-relieving medications.

Acupuncture is generally considered safe, as long as it is performed by a trained professional. When performed improperly, acupuncture can cause fainting, bleeding, and nerve damage and pose a risk for infection. For these reasons, you should always talk with your doctor or nurse beforehand, especially if you may have low white blood cell counts or thrombocytopenia from chemotherapy, to make sure that acupuncture can be performed in the safest manner possible. Acupressure is a variation of acupuncture in which the therapist presses on acupoints with her or his fingers rather than using needles.

Massage Therapy

In massage therapy, the therapist uses his or her hands or instruments (such as rollers) to manipulate, rub, and knead the body's muscles and soft tissue. Massage can be a useful adjunct to conventional medical treatments. Massage therapy can decrease stress, anxiety, depression, and pain while providing a temporary feeling of well-being and relaxation. Massage therapy may also be useful for relieving joint pain and stiffness, increasing mobility, rehabilitating injured muscles, stimulating nerves, increasing blood flow, and helping the circulation of the lymph system. Massage therapy should be conducted by a trained and licensed professional. You should always consult with your doctor or nurse before undergoing any type of therapy, particularly if you have a chronic condition such as arthritis or heart disease, to make sure that it is safe.

Transcutaneous Electrical Nerve Stimulation

Transcutaneous electrical nerve stimulation (TENS) is a CAM therapy used for pain relief in which a device transmits electric impulses through electrodes to an area of the body. A TENS system consists of an electric generator connected to pair of electrodes, which are attached to the skin near the area of pain and carry a mild electric current. A treatment session may last between five and fifteen minutes, and treatments can be applied as often as necessary. TENS may be administered by a physical therapist or applied at home using a portable TENS system.

Although TENS has been advocated for relief of both acute and chronic pain, most evidence indicates that it is most appropriate for short-term pain relief. Some cancer patients with mild pain related to nerve damage may benefit from TENS for brief periods of time. However, TENS will not cure the underlying causes of pain. Electrodes should not be placed over the eyes, heart, or brain, and people with heart problems should not use TENS.

Commonly Used Herbs

Echinacea

There are several kinds of echinacea (also known as Kansas snakeroot, black sampson, and purple cone flower) that are believed to provide immune enhancement and improve resistance to flu-like illnesses and colds. However, there is little evidence that it helps to boost the immune system or increase resistance to cancer. Echinacea is an herb that grows primarily in the Great Plains and eastern North America as well as in Europe. It can be associated with allergic reaction, so women with a history of asthma or allergic rhinitis should exercise caution. Echinacea may also cause liver damage, so if you are taking medications that have liver toxicity—for example, amiodarone (used for heart rhythm problems), anabolic steroids, methotrexate, or ketoconazole—echinacea should be avoided. When taken for long periods, echinacea may actually suppress the immune system, so women with autoimmune disorders (HIV disease or multiple sclerosis, for example) or those undergoing surgery should not take this preparation.

Kava

Kava (also known as kava kava and kavalactones) is a member of the pepper family that grows as a large shrub and is native to many islands in the South Pacific. It is promoted for relief of nervousness, anxiety, stress, and insomnia. Kava has no direct impact on cancer growth; however, its ability to ease anxiety may improve the quality of life. Kava is available in capsules, tablets, powder, and cream. A safe dose has not been determined, although 100 mg to 200 mg per day is commonly recommended. Kava should not be taken for longer than three months, and there are several precautions that need to be observed. Kava may slow down motor reflexes and reduce judgment when driving and may cause extreme drowsiness when taken with anti-anxiety medications or alcohol. It has the potential to interact with anesthetics and therefore should not be taken if you are to undergo surgery. Heavy or long-term use may result in liver damage, so women with a history of liver disease should not use kava. Rarely, kava may cause a rash, decreased urination, numbness of the mouth, or gastrointestinal discomfort.

Ginkgo

Ginkgo (also known as ginkgo biloba) is an extract from the ginkgo tree from China, Japan, and Korea. It is promoted for tinnitus (ringing in the ears), dizziness, and motion sickness and is believed to improve memory. While some herbalists have suggested that a compound in ginkgo, called ginkgolide B, may counteract body chemicals thought to promote cancer growth, there is no scientific evidence to support this claim. Ginkgo can be taken in pill or liquid form, with a recommended dose of 120–240 mg per day for up to three months. Ginkgo may interfere with normal blood clotting and therefore should not be taken if you are undergoing surgery or taking certain medications (aspirin, nonsteroidal anti-inflammatory drugs, or anticoagulants). Mild side effects that may be associated with ginkgo include stomach upset, headache, and allergic skin reactions.

Ginseng

Ginseng is a perennial plant that grows in China, Korea, Japan, Russia, and the United States. The dried root is promoted as a remedy to provide energy to people who are fatigued and to improve concentration. It is also believed by some to prevent cancer, although this claim is not supported by solid scientific evidence. Ginseng can be taken as a powder, a capsule, or a tea. Ginseng can cause restlessness, insomnia, headaches, and hypertension. Because of its estrogen-like effects, ginseng may have adverse effects in women with breast cancer or ovarian cancer. You should discuss these issues with your doctor or nurse before taking this preparation. In addition, ginseng can alter normal blood clotting and should not be used if you are undergoing surgery or taking anticoagulants (blood thinners).

St. John's Wort

St. John's wort (also known as goatweed, amber, klamath weed, and kira) is a shrublike plant that is native to Asia, northern Africa, and Europe and is also cultivated in the United States. The bright yellow flowers of this plant are used in herbal remedies. St. John's wort is commonly used to treat mild to moderate depression, anxiety, and sleep disorders. An average dose is 300 mg taken three times a day for up to six weeks. Side effects are not common but may include dizziness, fatigue, gastrointestinal pain, a rash, and hypersensitivity to sunlight. St. John's wort may interfere with conventional medications, including Coumadin, digoxin (a heart medicine), antidepressants, anesthesia, and certain types of chemotherapy (for example, etoposide). You should consult with your doctor or nurse before taking St. John's wort, especially if you are taking any prescription medications or other herbal preparations.

Dietary Supplements

Vitamin C

Vitamin C (also known as ascorbic acid) is an essential vitamin that is found in citrus fruits (oranges, grapefruits, and lemons), strawberries, green leafy vegetables, potatoes, bell peppers, and broccoli. Vitamin C is an antioxidant, which means that it blocks the action of activated oxygen molecules (free radicals), which can damage cells. Many scientific studies have shown a connection between consuming a diet high in fruits and vegetables and reducing the risks of certain cancers. However, it is unclear whether consuming vitamin C supplements can also reduce cancer risk. Other claims about vitamin C that are under investigation include whether it can enhance the immune system, prevent cancer from spreading, and help the body heal after cancer surgery. The recommended daily allowance of vitamin C is 75 mg per day. The upper limit is 2,000 mg per day, with dosages over this amount possibly causing nausea, diarrhea, stomach cramps, and headaches. Vitamin C doses over 1,000 mg per day should probably be avoided during cancer treatments.

Vitamin A

Vitamin A is obtained in the diet from animal sources and from beta carotene in plant foods. It is essential for normal growth, bone development, maintenance of healthy skin and mucous membranes, and protection against infections of the respiratory, gastrointestinal, and urinary tract. Vitamin A has not been shown to prevent cancer from developing, although some studies suggest that certain closely related molecules, called retinoids, may inhibit cancer development. The best way to get vitamin A is to eat a well-balanced diet of fruits, vegetables, dairy products, and animal fats. The recommended daily allowance of vitamin A is 4,000 IU (2.4 mg) per day. High doses of vitamin A can cause nausea, diarrhea, loss of appetite, fatigue, and headaches.

Vitamin E

Vitamin E is essential to the body in forming normal cells and healthy red blood cells. Like vitamin C, vitamin E is an antioxidant, and some proponents claim that vitamin E can protect the body against cancer by strengthening the immune system. Others believe that high doses may interfere with the effectiveness of radiation therapy or chemotherapy. Vitamin E may protect against colorectal and prostate cancers; however, there is no evidence that it can significantly affect cancers that have already developed. The main dietary sources of vitamin E are vegetable oils, green leafy vegetables, nuts, cereals, whole-wheat products, and egg yolks. The recommended daily allowance of vitamin E from food is 15 mg per day, which can generally be obtained from a balanced diet. The upper limit from supplements is 1,000 mg per day. Excessive doses of vitamin E taken for long periods can cause stomach pain, nausea, and diarrhea. High doses of vitamin E can alter the body's absorption of vitamins A, D, and K and should be avoided if you are taking Coumadin, as vitamin E supplements may counteract its blood-thinning effect.

Folic Acid

Folic acid (also known as folate, folacin, and vitamin B complex) is a B-complex vitamin found in vegetables, beans, fruits, and whole grains. It helps in cell metabolism and is important for the development of blood cells. Scientific studies have shown a connection between lower levels of folic acid and colorectal cancer and possibly cancers of the breast, lung, and stomach; however, the amount of folic acid needed to lower the risk is unknown. The recommended daily allowance of folic acid is 400 micrograms per day, which can be obtained from supplements or from a diet rich in dark green leafy vegetables, citrus fruits, and fortified grain-based cereals. If taken in extremely high doses, folic acid can be associated with nausea, flatulence, decreased appetite, and increased seizure activity in persons with a seizure disorder. In addition, high doses of folate can interfere with the effectiveness of certain chemotherapy drugs (for example, methotrexate).

Selenium

Selenium is an essential mineral nutrient that shows promise for preventing the development and progression of cancer; however, additional research is needed to confirm these claims. Selenium is also thought to improve elasticity of body tissues, improve blood flow to the heart, and prevent abnormal blood clotting. Dietary sources of selenium include seafood, whole grains, cereals, and Brazil nuts. The human body needs only a very small amount of selenium (the recommended intake is 5.5 micrograms

Table 8.2. Terms Used to Describe Vitamin Supplement
Recommendations

RDA (recommended daily allowance)
Designed to provide a base for evaluating the diet of groups, not
individuals. The RDAs do not allow for factors that may alter vitamins and minerals in foods, and the optimal levels of RDA for
certain nutrients are controversial.

RDI (reference daily intakes)
Based on the RDA. Represent intakes to achieve.

UTL (upper tolerable limits)
The upper safe daily limit, for adults only. The UTL can be
thought of as the highest daily intake over a prolonged time that
poses no risk to members of a healthy population.

---

per day), and excessive doses can be toxic. Signs of selenium poi-
soning include vomiting, fatigue, and loss of hair, teeth, and nails.

Coenzyme Q10

Coenzyme Q10 (also known as CoQ10) is an enzyme that reg-
ulates chemical reactions in the body and is believed to be an
antioxidant. Coenzyme Q10 has been promoted as a treatment
for cancer and immune deficiencies, but these claims have yet
to be proved conclusively. Some research indicates that coenzyme Q10 may have some protective effects against heart damage related to chemotherapy (for example, the agent doxorubicin). Coenzyme Q10 can be obtained from a number of foods,
including mackerel, sardines, beef, soybeans, peanuts, and
spinach. Coenzyme Q10 can also be obtained in supplemental
form as tablets or capsules, with a usual dosage of 90 to 400 mg
per day. There are few side effects from coenzyme Q10, which
may include headache, fatigue, diarrhea, and skin reactions.

In the preceding sections we have provided a brief summary of
some of the more commonly encountered complementary and

Table 8.3 Precautions for the Use of Supplements or Herbs

1. Always tell your health care provider about any supplements or herbs you are using, even if you are taking them for another condition.

2. Natural does not mean safe.

3. Using supplements, herbs, and medications simultaneously may increase the risk for an interaction.

4. Herbal products are not standardized.

5. Do not exceed recommended does.

6. Herbs and supplements are not monitored for quality.

7. Contamination of herbs and supplements may occur during the manufacturing process.

8. When in doubt, do without.

9. Safety is more important than efficacy.

alternative therapies. From a practical perspective, the complementary methods of mind, body, and spirit, as well as physical healing and manual touch, are most helpful when used in addition to conventional treatments to lessen side effects from ovarian cancer treatment or provide a sense of overall well-being. We would again caution against the use of herbal remedies or dietary supplements as alternatives to conventional treatment for ovarian cancer, since most of these methods have not been shown in rigorous scientific studies to have cancer-fighting effects. (See Tables 8.2 and 8.3.)

CAM Therapy Resources

Many resources are available, but not all of them provide reliable information. The following resources are reliable and provide information about different types of CAM therapies.

American Cancer Society
1-800-ACS-2345
www.cancer.org

National Cancer Institute's Cancer Information Service
1-800-242-6237

National Institutes of Health–National Center for Complementary
and Alternative Medicine
1-888-644-6226
www.nccam.nih.gov

Center for Alternative Medicine Research and Education
Beth Israel Deaconess Medical Center
Boston, MA
617-632-7770
www.compmed.caregroup.org

Health World Online
Culver City, CA
www.healthy.net/indexNet.asp

National Medicines Comprehensive Database
Pharmacist's Letter
Stockton, CA
www.naturaldatabase.com

Review of Natural Products Facts and Comparisons
St. Louis, MO
1-800-223-0554
www.drugfacts.com

Richard and Hilda Rosenthal Center for Complementary and
Alternative Medicine
College of Physicians and Surgeons
Columbia University
New York, NY
212-543-9550
www.rosenthal.hs.columbia.edu

American Massage Therapy Association
820 Davis St.
Evanston, IL 60201
www.amtamassage.org

Chapter 9

Image Recovery

We know it is hard for a patient to look in the mirror and see someone looking back at her whom she doesn't recognize. The combination of the pallor that many women have right after surgery, the weight loss from disease or surgery, and the loss of eyebrows and hair may indeed present a stranger in the mirror. Yet ovarian cancer and its treatment affect more than a patient's physical self-image: they also insult one's image of health, well-being, and mortality. They are an affront to the Whole Image, not simply the Visual Image. In this chapter we want to focus on image recovery in a global sense—the image recovery that occurs once the treatments are done and the disease is considered to be controlled.

Recovery of the Visual Image

On a fairly predictable time line and in a fairly predictable way, most women who have had surgery and chemotherapy will regain the physical appearance they had before treatment.

Hair, Nails, and Skin

Of the various aspects of recovery of the visual self, hair is the one you have the least control over. Your hair, fingernails, and skin will grow back on their own, and there isn't much you need to do to make sure this happens—although there are some things you can do to help your hair, fingernails, and skin recover from the trauma of treatment.

Studies have shown that a fair amount can be done from a nutritional perspective to strengthen hair and keep it strong. Adequate nutrition, from both vitamin supplements and food sources of protein, will help your hair and skin recover and will make them stronger. The issue of nutrition and cancer therapy has already been discussed (please refer to Chapter 6).

One of the biggest problems that many of our patients complain of when their hair first starts to grow back is that the hair is "brittle." This is probably due to the effects of chemotherapy on the collagen in the new hair strands as they start to grow out of the follicles. To keep your hair pliable and make it less likely to break off in the early weeks of growing back, use hair conditioners generously. Most people with long hair (that includes Rick) know that conditioners do a couple of things. They help to keep moisture in and on the hair strand and in the small pores in the hair (you have seen this on TV) at the same time that they lubricate the surface so the strands are more easily separated while brushing or combing. Lubricated strands of hair are less likely to break when being brushed.

Patients are sometimes startled to see that the hair that grows back is quite different from the hair that fell out. "Softer" and "curlier" are the two most frequent comments we hear. Another is that the hair has grown back in a different color, even in women who did not dye their hair before they had chemotherapy. Many women are amazed that what was once predominantly gray hair now comes out darker. It is worth noting that the hair that first grows in isn't like the hair that is going to be there in a year's time. Don't get too upset (or excited) with what you first get, because it is likely to change.

From the perspective of cancer treatment, there is nothing wrong with coloring or bleaching the new short hair that is growing back, but here's a word to the wise: this hair is not as durable and resilient as your hair was before chemotherapy or as it will be later. Bleaching in particular, and coloring hair in general, is brutal to the new hair strands and follicles and can lead to significant breaks and subsequent thinning. Just be careful, and always share with your hairdresser your recent history so she or he can select gentler, though potentially more transient, hair coloration techniques.

Weight

With the combination of being inactive and not taking in enough calories, a person unfortunately ends up losing weight in a manner that leads to loss of lean body mass (muscle) before loss of fat. Not fair, is it? What this means is that a patient who has been both inactive and nutritionally depressed will have lost a disproportionate amount of muscle mass. The flip side is that a woman recovering from her ovarian cancer treatment needs more than just calories. Not only do you want to see the woman in the mirror whom you are used to; you would like to see her appearing vivacious and full of health. Appropriate and aggressive nutritional support, which we talked about in Chapter 6, is critical to put pounds back on. But so is exercise, and that is what the next section discusses.

Recovery of Function

As many of us know from personal experience, gaining weight isn't that hard: you have to take in more calories than you consume, preferably at the same time eating correctly, with the appropriate amount of protein, carbohydrates, fat, and essential vitamins and minerals. Regaining the three Big S's—Strength, Stamina, and Sensation—isn't quite so quick and easy. The degree and rate of recovery of the first two S's is directly related to how much effort is personally put forth and for how long.

Body Strength and Stamina

Strength and stamina are two different things: strength is the ability to lift or move a given weight, while stamina is how long and or how many times can you lift or move that weight. To regain strength and stamina, you have to have a plan—a plan that is reasonable, employable, enjoyable, and long-term. Start your exercise program by selecting something physical that you like to do, and do it relatively infrequently for a relatively short period of time. An example:

> Susan M. decided that she wanted to regain her strength by walking. She thought mall walking would be fun, as the weather was always well controlled (something that can be a problem outdoors in Maryland), and she could look in the store windows as she walked (to keep from being bored), plus she could reward herself with a special little something to eat from the food court when she was done with the stroll. She found a time of day she liked, one that worked for her (morning), and set a frequency and length of time she was going to walk (twice a week for twenty minutes). Slowly she lengthened the time of the walk by five-minute increments (don't set a distance, set a time!) and by number of days, changing only one of the two variables every week. The goal set, with the guidance of her doctor, was to be walking at a brisk pace (enough to noticeably elevate her heart rate) for forty to fifty minutes, five days a week. Because she had set a reasonable goal, she reached her goal gradually and successfully over a period of about two months and found that her walking had become a routine she enjoyed.

It is very important not to succumb to the temptation to exercise "too much too soon." At some point all athletes (and this is what you are going to be now that you have an exercise plan that you are going to stick to) cave in to this temptation. If you exercise too much or too fast or even too frequently, all you do is become sore and tired, and you lose the motivation to get out and exercise again. Remember two cardinal rules of exercise: first, be reasonable; and second, any exercise is better than none. Another way of stating it is that the only really bad exercise is no exercise, which of course is an oversimplification.

There is another well documented advantage of exercising: it makes you feel better. You've heard of the runner's high? This general sense of "wellness" isn't only the result of looking better and healthier or of obtaining or regaining strength and stamina. It is in no small part a result of the release of endorphins, those powerful little "feel good" chemicals that can be activated by various activities. Blood endorphins go up when we eat chocolate, have an orgasm, or receive a nice compliment. They also go up when certain medications (analgesics) and drugs of abuse (narcotics) are used.

The endorphin release that comes from exercising is a good thing in many ways—ways that transcend the "feel good" effects. There are positive effects on blood flow to the essential body structures, as well as improved liver and kidney function. And, unlike the endorphin release that comes from eating chocolate or using illicit drugs, you can't get too much exercise-induced endorphins. The downside of routinely introducing increased circulating levels of endorphins in your body through exercise is that when you *don't* exercise, the levels don't go up, and you can get a bit of "withdrawal" and feel a bit "down." So now you have one more reason to get out and get those muscles clanking and heart beating faster!

Sensation

The rate and degree of return of sensation is beyond your control. We discussed these issues in the chapter on chemotherapy side effects (Chapter 4), but it is worth reviewing a couple of points. Because of the reality of what happens to the nerves, sensation may be one of the last, if not the very last, normal function recovered after cancer treatment has been completed. And there are some sensations that will never be the same as they were before treatment. The most common is the sensation changes around an incision site; these changes are part of the effects of the nerve endings being cut. These nerves never completely grow back in a way that matches the pre-incision state, and therefore, if we were to use an extremely sensitive instrument to measure sensation, we could find areas of persistent lack of sensation. Fortunately, over a period of months, most of the sensation in the tissue around an incision will return.

The same is not true for chemotherapy-induced abnormalities. It can take a year or more before the sensation loss stabilizes and then starts to recover. During this period it is crucial to take some small but important steps to minimize the chance that you will injure your body and to keep the muscles of the hands and feet (which are the two most commonly affected sites) supple and strong. Avoiding injury requires some forethought, so let's think about it! If you have intact sensation in your hands and you reach for a hot pot on the stove, you will almost instantaneously draw your hand back and likely avoid getting burned. But if there are even a few seconds' delay before the sensation of heat is registered, you could hold the pot too long and get burned. We have seen this happen not only with hands but also with burns on the abdomen from heating pads (when a woman wasn't able to feel how hot the pad actually was), with mashed fingers and toes, and with cuts from using knives and from walking barefoot in areas with sharp objects that the foot couldn't sense. Here are a few tips that can help protect your hands and feet if you experience chemotherapy-induced peripheral neuropathy:

- Always use an insulated mitt to pick up anything that may be hot off the stove or out of the microwave.
- Don't test water temperature with your hands or feet. Use a simple thermometer available from any hardware store, and don't insert a finger or a toe in any substance that is warmer than 120°F. Buy a couple of thermometers, and leave one in the kitchen and one in the bathroom.
- Always keep your toes and feet covered. No open-toed sandals. Wear closed-toe and closed-heel house slippers. Going barefoot is really silly.

~ When the weather starts getting into the low thirties, wear lightweight gloves. Buy a couple extra pairs of cheap ones, because we can promise that you will lose them.

~ Always wear gardening gloves (leather, not cloth) when gardening.

~ Keep your hands and feet clean, manicured and pedicured, and lubricated.

~ If you have any area of redness or potential infection that lasts more than three days, call your doctor.

The bottom line and last word of wisdom regarding the recovery of sensation is this: be patient. For almost everyone, the vast majority of the losses will be recovered.

Chapter 10

Taking Care of Social Needs

No woman is an island, or so the saying goes. This is no more fully true than when she is dealing with a life-threatening disease like ovarian cancer. The people around you, including family, friends, and simply acquaintances, are affected, either actively or passively, to some extent by what is happening to you. In considering your social needs, this chapter looks at your relationships with other people, including your sexual relationships.

Family and Friends

We humans are tribal folks. We don't want to offend anyone, but we have to comment that living a physically and emotionally isolated life is inconsistent with how we humans evolved and were created. For example, when someone we know dies, we feel sadness at their passing, even if we didn't know them well. And similarly, even if we have never met the deceased person's spouse or children, we feel compassion for them in their inevitable suffering. These feelings of sadness and compassion illustrate the connections that exist between humans.

During times of either real or perceived crisis, family structures and interpersonal relationships are put to the test, and their strengths or weaknesses become evident. We have seen this happen so many times that we like to raise this issue with our patients as soon as the first shock of the ovarian cancer diagnosis has worn off. You really need to be proactive in your interactions with family and friends. This is definitely *not* a time just to let matters run their own course. You need to ask (and answer) very specific questions (some of these are discussed below). We encourage you to write the answers down. Appreciate that over the months and years of dealing with ovarian cancer, your answers to these questions probably will change. That's okay—in fact, it's preferable. There is a bias against individuals who, after thoughtful consideration, change their opinions about important matters, and we often belittle folks who do that. Don't share this bias, and in particular don't belittle yourself for changing your mind!

Here are some questions to think about when interacting with family and friends:

Who do I want to know that I have ovarian cancer? There are women who don't want anyone to know the truth about their ovarian cancer and the anticipated treatments. Among the patients who have felt this way in our own practices, their desire to keep matters secret is usually the result of one or more views. Some don't want to burden other folks with the worry that may come with sharing the diagnosis. Others are fearful that they will be treated "differently" in a negative way, either personally or professionally. And one or two patients just didn't think it was anybody's business but their own! Generally, though, you will want to tell the individuals you are the closest to, the people who you know will provide emotional as well as practical help.

What do I want people to know? Once the decision has been made to share what is going on, you have to decide how much you want those around you to know. Realize that people are going to figure out that something significant is happening, especially because of the visible changes associated with chemotherapy and the occasional limitations in your ability to do things you usually do. We have encouraged our patients to choose a select core of individuals whom they are the closest to, the people they are most likely to rely on for emotional and physical assistance, and pretty much tell them everything. As humans we have a desire to know, and we can make up data to fill in the holes in what we know, usually coming up with something worse than the truth. Also remember that we are tribal and that people do genuinely care about what is happening to you. That care and concern can come from some of the least expected sources.

A patient of Rick's, Carol B., lived away from her immediate family and had not yet established close friendships, so she was quite isolated. Carol didn't know it, but the woman living next door had lost her mother to cancer. During the time of the neighbor's mother's treatment and eventual death, there had been some estrangement, and the neighbor suffered guilt about how little she had been able to help her mother during her sickness. In a casual conversation at the elevator, the neighbor commented that she hadn't seen Carol for a while. Carol, who had been in the hospital, shared only the most superficial facts of what had been going on with her ovarian cancer and treatments. The neighbor asked if there was something she could do to help, particularly in light of the neighbor's knowledge about what cancer treatment can be like. To make a long story short, because the neighbor worked evening hours, she was able to become a great transportation resource as well as a "security net" for Carol. But the most wonderful thing about the whole story is that the neighbor, in her ability to help Carol, was personally rewarded and able to resolve what had transpired with her own mother. Carol unwittingly gave much more in sharing her ovarian cancer experience than she ever received.

The moral of Carol's story is not that you should set up a Web site and provide blow-by-blow reports on your treatments, or do mass mailings. But at the same time, don't be selfish: share what is happening in your life with those whom you even casually deal with. You are doing them a service.

What sort of old, unresolved issues and difficulties are going to arise when I start dealing with my family and friends? Forewarned is definitely forearmed, and this is something that you will want to anticipate. Even in the most "functional" of families there are prior experiences and "track records" of behavior that may need to be re-addressed or at least remembered. Think about what these issues may be, but don't spend a lot of time trying to resolve issues from prior unpleasant experiences or failed interactions. All interpersonal interactions have a prior history that colors today's experiences. But this history doesn't or shouldn't dictate what happens today. Gloriously, we are capable of infinite change and revival.

We have been known to become involved when family members of our patients won't let old issues rest. For example, Rick says: "As a person who has dedicated his life to caring for women with cancer, there is little that irritates me more than seeing all this 'baggage' being brought up from the emotional cellar. Some patients of mine have suffered to a much greater degree from their family interactions during the ovarian cancer treatments then they ever did from the diagnosis and treatment of the ovarian cancer itself. In these settings I must admit that I may have overstepped my bounds, but, in my perceived role as the ultimate advocate, I have told the family to get over it, stop emotionally torturing my patient, and just leave her alone! And there are times when the family members will start at each other, too. Oh my goodness.

"Not being a family counselor, I strongly encourage these families to undergo therapy, and I formally recommend that they do so, giving them the names and numbers of counseling centers. However, I always advocate strongly for my patient, and at times I will almost in a paternalistic way protect my patient from the family. There are more than a few members of families of my patients who don't care much for me because of the protective and advocacy stance that I take with my patients. To tell you the truth, I don't really care, because my patients are almost universally grateful when I play this role."

In summary, think about what you want to tell to whom, and be prepared for what your family may do. If matters get tough with family or friends, the effort spent in formal counseling is usually worthwhile.

Sexuality

Wonderfully, we are sexual beings to our very core. Whether you believe that we were created this way or evolved this way doesn't matter. It is just the way we are. And though there are many members of society who for personal or religious reasons choose the celibate life, they are few and their rationale for doing so is really not our concern. Yet even those individuals who have cho sen celibacy are still sexual beings.

Sometimes it amazes us how weird our society has been about sex, its role and performance. We're not going to go on a rant, but we do want to share our general views about the role of sexuality in people's lives, so you can understand where our opinions come from. We believe that sexual function serves three purposes (in order of priority): procreation, intimacy and bonding, and fun. Now you can argue that one or all of these are not justifiable and that the order is incorrect, but if you believe that the obligation to procreate is essential, we think our order of priority makes sense.

Related views that we hold, which have to do with how sexuality is manifested, are that sex must never be a weapon, that it must be freely consensual, and that it must never be used to manipulate. We believe that one of the reasons there has been so much fear by certain societies or sections of societies about sex is that it can be a powerful destructive force if applied as a weapon or used to manipulate. But so can love . . .

There are natural changes in the frequency of sexual per formance that occur with both the aging of individuals and the aging of a relationship. Most of us can remember the sexual intensity of a new relationship. Fortunately for some of us that intensity not only continues but deepens over time, but the frequency of the sexual acts usually doesn't increase. That is unfortunate, because there is something just wonderfully otherworldly about the intimacy that occurs, the bonds that are strengthened, by the physical closeness of sexual encounters. This doesn't necessarily mean that orgasm occurs for either or both of the partners. Sexuality is much, much more than that. It is a feeling of completeness and part of what makes us whole. That is why we are such strong advocates for sexual encounters for patients who may be having chunks of their vision of "wholeness" removed. To quote the TV ads: "It's healthy and fun!"

Sexual Desire and Responsiveness: Often a woman who is either undergoing treatment for ovarian cancer or recovering from treatment will comment that she just doesn't understand why she isn't responsive to her partner's sexual approaches. "I don't love him (or her) any less, but I am just not interested. What is happening to me?" We try to explain in a relatively direct fashion something that is multifaceted and complex: the human libido.

Sexual desire and responsiveness are a product of multiple different things. Unquestionably, there is a hormonal component. We know that the ovaries of a reproductive-age woman produce a small amount of androgens. These androgens belong to the same family of sex steroids as testosterone, and we all know what testosterone does to sexual appetite and drive. Just walk into the room of any adolescent American male, and you can pretty much feel the sex drive, though it is remarkably disorganized and not uncommonly poorly directed. As a woman gets older and enters the latter part of her reproductive life, her sex steroid levels will become lower. This occurs to a greater degree with the estrogen compounds than with the androgenic compounds (the ones that are biochemically related to sexual drive and appetite).

Being diagnosed with, receiving treatment for, and recovering from ovarian cancer cause a wide range of physical, biochemical, and emotional changes that can affect a woman's libido. Restoring libido to a level that is satisfactory to the patient requires an understanding of the complex interplay between all of these factors. Many times, image-enhancement techniques can help restore a woman's sense of well-being and self-confidence. A consultation between the patient, her partner, and a professional sex therapist may also be of benefit in helping the partner learn (or relearn) how to help the patient herself "feel attractive" during treatment and after completing treatment. In addition, both hormonal and nonhormonal medications can be prescribed to increase a woman's libido. It is advisable to have an open-ended discussion with your doctor about these issues, so that each of your needs can be addressed adequately.

Chapter 11

Recurrent Disease

Unfortunately, many women with ovarian cancer have to deal with recurrence of their disease. Depending upon the initial stage of disease at the time of diagnosis, as few as 5 percent and as many as 70 percent of women who have been treated for ovarian cancer have a recurrence. The numbers regarding the outcomes of primary treatment of ovarian cancer are far from what we want for our patients: about 55 percent of all women with ovarian cancer end up facing recurrent disease, and except in the most unusual situations, the recurrence leads to a fatal outcome.

Many patients are startled to find out that a "gold standard" for the management of recurrent ovarian cancer doesn't exist, as it does for the management of newly diagnosed or suspected ovarian cancer, although there are general guidelines that are commonly followed (these guidelines are discussed in this chapter). From our perspective, there are several reasons for the lack of a "gold standard" or uniform approach to treatment of women with recurrent disease (or, to put it another way, there are several reasons why a tailor-made approach to treatment must be created for each individual patient):

1. The probability of response to a second-line therapy is directly related to the time interval between the completion of the initial therapy and the diagnosis of the recurrence.
2. The unique desires of the patient, always dominant, are paramount when dealing with a now incurable disease. Many in-

dividuals are willing to put up with a significant deterioration in quality of life if they think they have a chance of being cured. The willingness to do the same in the setting of a probably fatal outcome varies greatly from patient to patient.

3. Because toxicity from therapy is to some degree additive with each subsequent treatment the patient receives, prior chemotherapy toxicity and residual impairment from chemotherapy toxicity must be taken into consideration when devising a treatment regimen for each patient.

4. There is growing evidence that we can predict which patients will respond to which chemotherapy by using what is called *in vitro testing* (something we discuss below). If cancer cells have been harvested, and if these cancer cells can be grown and tested in the laboratory, the information gained may be of great value in selecting a patient-specific therapy.

The General Principle: Start Again

Remember this phrase: "Start again." Start again with determining the extent of disease. Start again with the discussion of options and decision-making processes. Start again with a surgical approach. Start again with chemotherapy.

Of course, nothing in medicine is that simple, and in fact options and decisions in the treatment of recurrent disease are greatly influenced by the woman's previous treatment and the rest of her medical history. So we are not really starting at the beginning again, but we are going through the processes again, informed by what has gone on previously.

As noted above, there are general guidelines for the treatment of recurrent disease; these guidelines are presented here.

Confirmation of Disease

The first thing that needs to be done when there is a concern that ovarian cancer may have recurred is to confirm whether it really has recurred. How intensely we search for confirmation and how certain we can be about what's true depends, of course, on what steps the patient wants to take to find out whether the cancer has recurred. Most patients don't want to decide what to do about recurrence, however, until there is a definitive confirmation of disease recurrence. Therefore it is important for the patient to have a thorough physical examination, blood tests, a battery of imaging studies, and other tests. Biopsies of suspicious lesions are commonly made, unless radiographic and laboratory findings are definitive, in which case there is no question about the nature of the disease and therefore no reason to expose the patient to any risk of biopsy.

Time Interval to Recurrence

Once we are convinced of the recurrent nature of the disease, the next thing to determine is how much time elapsed between the time when the patient was believed to be disease-free and the time when the disease recurred. The shorter the time interval, the less likely it is that the disease will respond to any chemotherapy, even if we try new agents. Sometimes it is difficult to pin down the time of "last evidence of disease" or when a patient entered into "remission." We generally use the date of the last cycle of the front-line chemotherapy, but other health care providers may use the last date on which there was any biochemical, physical, or radiographic evidence of disease, if this evidence was gathered before the initial chemotherapy was finished. The majority of the scientific literature supports the belief that if the disease-free interval is less than six months, then re-treatment with the initial drugs (usually carboplatin and Taxol) is not likely to work. The drugs that should be used for these patients are discussed below.

Surgery

We also use that six-month criterion in deciding whether to seriously consider *secondary cytoreductive surgery* (that is, a second surgery similar to the first, undertaken with the goal of removing one or more tumors). In general, if a patient's disease recurs within six months, she won't be asked if she wants a secondary cytoreductive surgery unless (a) we are not sure that the first surgery was a sincere and skilled attempt at aggressive initial cytoreductive surgery or (b) the patient wants the second surgery very much and has an overwhelming reason to undergo a relatively low-gain and real-risk procedure. For example, a woman in her thirties or forties who has young children might well fit in this second category.

To our disappointment and surprise, we see a remarkable number of women whose initial surgeries may not have been optimal, although the majority have had cytoreductive surgery at some time during their initial therapy regimen, either as interval cytoreductive surgery or at the time of a proposed "second look." For a woman who may not have had optimal initial surgery, we will reevaluate her situation and attempt the initial cytoreductive surgery; functionally, we will treat the patient as if she had never been operated on. This means that we don't have rules about how many lesions show up on the patient's imaging studies, though we are careful to determine the patient's "performance" status (general health and ability to care for herself) and her wishes. We know that the fewer lesions that are detected before the surgery or that are evident at the time of surgery, the more likely it is that we can remove all of the recurrent disease and that the patient will benefit from the surgery.

Certain observations about cytoreductive surgery and ovarian cancer are inherently true no matter where the patient is in her own ovarian cancer history. We outlined these in Chapter 2. Some of these truths are worth restating: first, the less cancer you have at the completion of the surgery, the more likely it is that you will get a meaningful and long disease-free survival. Furthermore, if the surgery cannot reduce the lesions to a size less than 2 centimeters in diameter (the diameter of a dime), the surgery will not have made a difference in your survival. Associated with this latter truth is another: if it is known that there is no reasonable chance of removing, or "debulking," the lesions so that they are less than 2 centimeters, there really should not be any attempt at surgery. Secondary cytoreductive surgery carries a 15 to 25 percent risk of a significant life-threatening complication and about a 1 percent chance of death.

Although we don't follow any hard and fast rules, when patients have more than six to ten distinct areas that are highly suspicious for or are confirmed as recurrent disease, we will usually not offer an attempt at secondary cytoreductive surgery. We certainly would not offer an attempt when the radiographic findings are consistent with "miliary" disease (disease in which "seeds" of cancer are widely dispersed), or when the disease is located in places that cannot be resected (operated on). However, if there is isolated disease in places that are difficult to resect, we will still attempt surgery, recruiting the specialized surgical assistance (hepatobiliary, thoracic, vascular, and so on) that we may need in order to make the best attempt at resection using the most skilled and experienced hands available.

Every patient who is considering secondary cytoreductive surgery must remember that the risk of suffering a major complication either during or after the operation is quite real. For some women, either they or we feel that the risk is just too high. Patients must always be informed of the potential for complications as well as the potential for benefit before they decide whether to go ahead with a given treatment or procedure.

Chemotherapy

Almost all women who have recurrence of ovarian cancer will receive some form of *second-line chemotherapy* or *salvage chemotherapy*. The question is, Which agent should be recommended? There are a few facts that help us determine which chemotherapy to offer. Some of these we mentioned earlier, but here is a list of them all together:

1. Time interval from completion of front-line therapy to recurrence.
2. Toxicity from initial therapy.

3. Results of specific laboratory tests called *clonogenic assays*.
4. Risk for toxicity from the proposed salvage chemotherapy.

Let's talk about each one of these.

Time Interval from Completion of Front-Line Therapy to Recurrence. As previously stated, if ovarian cancer recurs within six months after the completion of front-line therapy, it is unlikely to respond meaningfully to the drugs that were first administered. Therefore we generally not only use different drugs but sometimes even avoid administering drugs that are from the same family (for example, we usually would not give cisplatin to a woman who had previously received carboplatin). Like pretty much everything associated with recurrent ovarian cancer, this is not a hard and fast rule. But in general, women who have been treated with the conventional carboplatin and Taxol combination will not be re-treated with those drugs. They will usually receive either topotecan, Doxil, or some other approved drug, depending upon the variables listed below.

Toxicity from Initial Therapy In Chapter 4, on chemotherapy-related side effects, we explained that every drug regimen has its own toxicity profile. In addition, every woman being treated for ovarian cancer has her own response to any given regimen. Therefore, it is critically important to obtain very thorough information, not only about side effects (neuropathy, persistent bone marrow suppression, renal dysfunction, and so on) that may persist, but also about all side effects that occurred, even if they have gone away. When we are selecting a second-line treatment (or third or fourth, and so on), if we have a choice, we will not give a regimen that has the same type of side effects or potential toxicity as the former treatment regimen had. Again, this is not a hard and fast rule, but it is one that we generally follow.

If a woman's ovarian cancer recurs after a long time interval, it may also be that she has developed new medical problems unrelated either to her ovarian cancer or to the chemotherapy she received. These problems may affect treatment, and so a complete medical history is always needed and must be updated frequently.

Results of Clonogenic Assays. At the time of secondary cytore-ductive surgery, we will do a sterile collection of tissue that can be grown and tested in a laboratory in an attempt to determine which chemotherapy agent may be the most logical, if not the best, choice. There are multiple for-profit corporations that offer this testing service, each of them claiming that its test is better than or offers advantages over its competitors'. Which company performs the study doesn't matter, as this testing works much the same way in all of them. The important thing to remember is that the result of this kind of test is better at predicting what *won't* work than what *will* work.

Clonogenic assays are done this way: once the tissue is re-moved from the body, a pathologist is called into the operating room immediately to collect the specimen. Maintaining sterile technique, the pathologist takes the specimen to the pathology department, where representative parts are collected on which to perform traditional evaluation. Then at least a gram of cancer tissue (about the size of the end of your little finger) is packed in dry ice and sent via overnight delivery to the commercial lab-oratory. The laboratory processes the specimen and grows the cells in test tubes (*in vitro*), in the environment of both differ-ent drugs and different drug combinations, and in different con-centrations of the drugs. These samples provide information about which drugs the cancer is more or less likely to respond to.

These technologies have some significant limitations, how-ever. First, a large number of cells must be harvested. If a woman with recurrent ovarian cancer has a needle biopsy, there is no way enough cells will be available to get a meaningful growth. Second, the cancer cells have to grow. This is no small feat, since in up to 40 percent of the cases the cells won't grow in the arti-ficial environment that is the laboratory. Third, the testing is much better at predicting what the cancer cells will *not* respond to than it is in predicting whether a drug will kill the cancer cells growing in the patient. We use the clonogenic assays as much to choose which drugs not to use as to decide which drugs to use.

There is growing information from increasingly large studies that confirm the value of selecting not only second- but also front-line therapy using in vitro sensitivity testing. It is imperative that the patient understand, though, that selecting front-line therapy using this testing must be considered nothing other than experimental.

Risk for Toxicity from the Proposed Salvage Chemotherapy. Every drug has its own associated side effects, which we call *toxicity.* Most of these side effects, as we discussed earlier in this book, are transient, but many will have some degree of residual effects. The residual effects can be as silent as a chronic suppression of the bone marrow's ability to produce white cells or as obvious as a peripheral neuropathy that interferes with such simple tasks as buttoning a blouse. The toxicity that has occurred before is predictive of what toxicity will occur later—that is, the doctor needs to know what kind of toxicity the patient previously experienced so he or she can counsel the patient about what toxicity she may have with the second or subsequent therapies.

In addition, any other symptoms that are a result of ongoing medical problems may get worse when chemotherapy is administered. And when ovarian cancer recurs, the patient has naturally become older, and any symptoms of other diseases or conditions will probably have become more significant or remarkable. Therefore, when we are selecting a different type of chemotherapy, we strongly emphasize the importance of previous toxicities. If we are considering equally effective therapies and one has a toxicity that is not the same as those the patient has previously suffered or has residual effects from, we select that therapy.

Investigational Protocols

Women being treated for ovarian cancer are most likely to be treated on an investigational protocol when the disease has recurred. Therefore, although we discussed investigational protocols extensively in Chapter 3, we want to say more about them here.

Because there is no "standard" chemotherapy that should be used when ovarian cancer returns, theoretically, any time a woman with recurrent ovarian cancer is treated, it is an "investigation." But what we really mean by *investigation* is either (1) that drugs that have been shown to work and that have been approved by the FDA will be studied ("investigated") in different dosages, combinations, or routes of administration, and the outcomes will be compared to each other, or (2) that new drugs that have not been proven or for which the best dose is not known will be evaluated.

We strongly believe in offering patients the option of participating in investigational studies as soon as the patients are eligible. There are numerous advantages, but for the patient with recurrent disease, there is none in our opinion more important than the opportunity to try new drugs. The big risk, of course, is that the treatment won't work at all and the ovarian cancer will grow unencumbered. For us there is not a lot of concern regarding this risk, because we keep remarkably close tabs on our patients (as do all investigators). If there is any sign that the therapy is not working, the treatment is stopped and a conventional, approved drug can be substituted. We can always give a different approved drug.

But we cannot always switch to investigational drugs. The "rules of enrollment" are such that a patient who has received three or more "treatment regimens" (meaning drugs or combinations of drugs) may not be able to be treated on an investigational protocol. The only real concern, from our perspective, is that the patient will develop side effects from the investigational drug that will make it impossible for her to receive conventional drugs, or that she won't be able to tolerate conventional drugs. This is a risk we take.

If you are reading this book and have recurrent disease, we strongly encourage you to talk to your oncologist about receiving investigational drugs in a study protocol. There is an inaccurate belief that to receive any investigational drug, a patient has to be treated at a major academic institution or cancer center. That just isn't true. Both the National Cancer Institute and pharmaceutical companies sponsor investigations that are performed in community cancer centers like the ones in which the majority of readers are being treated. The only way you will find out is by asking, so do just that: Ask!

Complementary and Alternative Therapies

There are so many books and Web sites out there that talk about so many complementary and alternative therapies. Vitamins, herbs, supplements, teas—the list goes on and on. Chapter 8 covers all these therapies in detail. Here we provide some general guidelines on *ingested alternative therapies* (which do not include relaxation, meditation, and other therapies that are not taken by mouth or injection) for our patients with recurrent disease.

Let the Buyer Beware

The companies that make these products are out to make a profit. There is nothing wrong with that: it's the American way! Unfortunately, however, fantastic claims often are made based on absolutely no data. Yet the manufacturers know that people with terminal disease sometimes become desperate and may be willing to spend their last dollar trying to lengthen their life in a meaningful way, even if the proposed treatment has no scientific basis. Many of these therapies are expensive—some are quite expensive—and most are totally unregulated: they are sold as vitamins or nutritional supplements, not as medications, at whatever price the market will bear. Be careful.

Don't Let the Alternative Therapy Interfere with Medical Therapy

Many patients believe that it is either one or the other: either do what my doctor recommends or use these alternative therapies. That is just not the case! We look at what most people consider "alternative therapies" and label them "complementary," meaning that they aren't used *instead of* but rather *along with* regular medical therapies. This leads to the next point . . .

Make Sure Your Doctor Knows What You Are Taking

Every time we see a patient, we ask her what medications she is taking. After she has answered, we ask, "Are you taking anything else?" We want to know the truth, not because we are going to tell her to stop taking the alternative medications, but so we can make sure she isn't taking anything that is known to be toxic or to have the potential for a serious interaction with any standard medication she is taking. Here's an example.

In the late 1980s and early 1990s, shark cartilage was popular as an alternative cancer therapy in certain parts of the country. It was not known whether it worked (despite the fantastic claims by the marketers), and it was also not known whether it had a significant toxicity. What researchers found out—and this was reported in the medical literature—was that shark cartilage significantly decreased the levels of platelets (the cells that help stop bleeding) in certain patients. Carboplatin and Taxol, two drugs that are front-line therapy for ovarian cancer, also decrease platelet levels, and a woman taking one of these drugs and also taking shark cartilage might well have increased side effects and experience increased toxicity. This might make it impossible for the patient to take the full dose of treatment and could even cause a significant life-threatening hemorrhage (bleeding). Because studies showed that shark cartilage had no effect on the common cancer cell types, what a woman got was all risk and no benefit!

The bottom line is, if your doctor doesn't know what you are taking, how can she or he warn you about potential "drug interactions"? Please tell your doctor if you are taking or considering taking any alternative or complementary therapies.

Radiation Therapy

Radiation therapy, in our opinion and in the opinion of our associates of the Kelly Gynecologic Oncology Service at the Johns Hopkins Hospital and Medical Institutions, has no role in the front-line therapy of women with ovarian cancer. It does play some limited part in the management of select women with recurrent disease. To reiterate what we said in Chapter 5, the problem with radiation therapy is not that it doesn't work; it is that in the majority of cases it kills or injures normal cells to such a degree that it just isn't worth it.

We utilize radiation therapy in two specific settings. In the order of probability that we would recommend the treatment, those settings are (1) an isolated site of recurrence that has been totally or almost totally resected and (2) unresectable local disease causing a significant, though probably not fatal, complication.

Isolated Site of Recurrence

Radiation therapy is effective at killing low numbers (small volumes) of ovarian cancer. It isn't able to sterilize any tumor nodule that is much larger then 3 to 5 millimeters (about the size of the nonaction end of a pen), but it can *shrink* much larger nodules. We often use radiation therapy for a woman who has an isolated (meaning one) recurrence that has been either totally resected or resected so that there is only minimal (1-millimeter) disease left. At the completion of the resection, we will mark the site of resection with titanium clips, placing three clips each at the top, bottom, left, and right edges. With the help of a CT scan port, the patient will then receive a limited field of radiation, with doses ranging up to 50 Gray, depending upon the specific site of the disease and the patient's ability to tolerate the treatment. Although this treatment is generally not curative, in some select cases it will be, and in many settings it can gain the patient significant time and control of symptoms.

Unresectable Local Disease

Some women with recurrent ovarian cancer develop a dominant site of metastasis that is not responsive to chemotherapy and not easily resected without a high probability of a significant complication. A classic example is a woman with a group of matted lymph nodes in the area of the scalene anticus fat pad (the base of the neck on the left side). These nodes can be unsightly and painful and can lead to significant symptoms as a result of compression on nerves or the major blood vessels that supply or drain the left arm. It is unlikely that a patient will die from this potentially disabling site of recurrence, although in extremely rare cases the malignancy erodes into the blood vessels, leading to a fatal hemorrhage.

Local radiation therapy is a valuable option in the management of this isolated and potentially, if not actually, symptomatic site of recurrence. The radiation therapy probably does not prolong life, though it has a very reasonable chance of increasing the quality of life.

Hormonal Therapy

The term *hormonal therapy* is a catch phrase for a whole group of treatment options. These options include progesterones (one of the two dominant naturally occurring sex steroids that are produced mostly by the premenopausal ovary), anti-estrogens (tamoxifen, raloxifene), aromatase inhibitors (Arimidex, among others), and antigonadotropin therapy.

Progesterones

Progesterone is the "second female sex steroid." During a woman's reproductive life, progesterone is produced in the ovary, after each ovulation occurs (the monthly release of an egg that is ready to be fertilized by sperm). Progesterone is the dominant hormone in the second half of the menstrual cycle (days 15 through 28 of a 28-day cycle), with the highest levels of progesterone being produced around day 21 or so. It is progesterone that complements and to some degree counteracts the effects of estrogen on the lining of the uterus (the endometrium), first by making the endometrium ready to receive the fertilized egg, and second by inhibiting, when there are adequate progesterone levels, the carcinogenic effects of estrogen.

Progesterone has been shown to have some limited effect in the management of selected cases of metastatic endometrial cancer. It has not been shown to be effective against recurrent ovarian cancer. That said, progesterone, as a result of its appetite-inducing and weight-gaining effects, may be useful in managing some of the side effects related to ovarian cancer treatment.

Anti-Estrogens

Tamoxifen and its sister component raloxifene are proven and highly effective therapies for a large number of women with the most common hormonally related malignancy in American women: breast cancer. Although it is not completely understood how these so-called selective estrogen receptor modulators (SERMs) work, we do know that they seem to block the estrogen receptor so that it is not able to respond to strong estrogenic stimulation. The SERMs have some effect in the treatment of recurrent ovarian cancer, but the rates or responses are not even close to those reported when SERMs are used in the treatment of estrogen-receptor-positive breast cancer. Reported response rates in recurrent ovarian cancer are in the range of 12 to 15 percent at best. Even though these numbers are not very encouraging, for some women who have suffered significant toxicity from prior cytotoxic chemotherapy and who wish to do something, while not exposing themselves to major side effects, tamoxifen may be an option.

Aromatase Inhibitors

The major source of estrogens in postmenopausal women is not the ovaries. Instead, postmenopausal women have a weak estrogen called *estrone* that is produced by *peripheral conversion*. What happens is that the adrenal glands produce a hormone called *androstendione*. Androstendione is actually an androgen (one of the so-called male hormones). The androstendione is "peripherally converted" by the adipocyte (fat cell) to estrone. The enzyme that is necessary to make this conversion is called *aromatase*. A relatively new generation of drugs called the *aromatase inhibitors* block this enzyme, stopping the conversion of androstendione to estrone and leading to even a lower total amount of circulating biologically active estrogens.

The aromatase inhibitors have proved to be a useful therapy for women with hormonally sensitive breast cancers whose cancer is no longer responsive to the SERMs or who cannot tolerate the SERMs because of the associated side effects. There are multiple aromatase inhibitors that have been approved by the FDA; the differences between them may be of more commercial importance than patient-care significance. To date, however, there is little experience with the use of aromatase inhibitors in the management of recurrent ovarian cancer. One can anticipate that the response rates should be no better than what is seen with the SERMs and that only ovarian cancers that are estrogen sensitive (those that have been proved to express or are likely to express the estrogen receptor) will respond to aromatase inhibitor therapy.

Antigonadotropins

Follicle-stimulating hormones called *gonadotropins* (also spelled *gonadotrophins*) stimulate the ovaries to produce and release eggs and to produce the sex steroids (estrogen and progesterone) that make the uterus receptive to the fertilized egg. When a woman goes through menopause, whether surgically or as a natural part of aging, she produces significantly less estrogen and progesterone. Sensing this decrease in hormone production, the brain produces gonadotropins, to make the ovary work harder. Unfortunately, when the ovaries are absent, there are no ovaries to respond to the increased "push" produced by the high levels of gonadotropins. And even when a woman still has ovaries, once she has been through menopause, her ovaries are no longer as responsive to gonadotropins as they once were. The woman with ovarian cancer will have high circulating gonadotropin levels.

It has been documented that many ovarian cancer cells possess what is called the *gonadotropin receptor*, and it has been proposed that the circulating high levels of gonadotropins in a woman who is postmenopausal or who has had her ovaries removed may serve to stimulate ovarian cancer cell growth, at a very low but constant level. It would make sense to consider blocking these gonadotropins as a way of influencing ovarian cancer cell growth. Although this is a good theory and there are some excellent data to support these assumptions, we don't yet know if all the assumptions behind the theory are true.

A drug called Lupron, which blocks the production of the gonadotropins, is widely used in treating nonmalignant diseases such as endometriosis and fibroids that are estrogen responsive, as well as prostate cancer. The drug works by making people either hypoandrogenic or hypoestrogenic (low androgen levels or low estrogen levels), depending upon whether the patient is female or male. Lupron has been studied as a treatment for recurrent ovarian cancer and yields response rates similar to those achieved with the anti-estrogens (12 to 15%).

At the beginning of this chapter we introduced the concept of "starting again" in managing recurrent ovarian cancer. This approach means that the treatment approach should be based on the current situation but interpreted within the context of the patient's prior therapy, current life goals, general health, and ability to tolerate the proposed new therapy. In other words, treatment should be individualized and based on one or more of the therapeutic options discussed above. Newer treatments for recurrent ovarian cancer, such as gene therapy and immunotherapy, are currently being developed and will, we hope, expand the available choices for successfully managing recurrent disease.

Chapter 12

Decisions at the End of Life

An anecdote from Rick provides one perspective on the value of self-determination as a person approaches the end of life: "Recently my sixteen-year-old son, Rocky, and I saw a movie that was the most popular movie in America the week it was released. The movie lacked plot and character development, but it was great adolescent-boy entertainment and almost worth the seventeen dollars I had to pay for us to get in. There was one line in the flick that was worth remembering and, believe it or not, is quite appropriate to mention in this chapter. Two action-hero brothers are off to engage in righteous battle. Before they charge into the horde of bad guys, they look each other in the eye and scowl, 'Live free, die well.' Pretty trite, huh? And, I think most of us would also say, not a bad motto to live and die by."

We are not going to address the issue of living free, though that wouldn't be a bad topic for an entire book about how to deal with cancer. But we do need to spend some time talking about dying well. The discussion is divided into two sections, one on end-of-life decisions (this chapter) and the other on death (the next chapter). From a time-line perspective, we will talk about what happens from the time a disease becomes incurable to the time the heart and lungs stop—when a medical professional would be willing to verify death. Just as we are going to avoid the issue of what it means to live free, we are going to avoid a big discussion about when someone actually dies, though probably we all have our own opinions about when that is.

In this chapter we focus on how patients make decisions about what happens up until the terminal event and thereafter. For a discussion of the issues that can be controlled in and around the moment of death, see Chapter 13.

Here's a story from Rick's own experience that illustrates the importance of an open dialogue between the patient and her caregivers when treatment options have run out:

Not long ago I had to do one of the most painful and at the same time one of the most personally rewarding things that I do as a cancer doc. I had to keep a promise to Dana F. and share with her, one of my long-time patients, the reality that despite all I had tried to do for her, we really had run out of options. Curing her disease had long ago fallen away as a potential option. And now, even our ability to meaningfully prolong her life had evaporated.

When I first met Dana three years before, she was a healthy and active professional woman who was director of sales for a large national organization. She was married to a great guy, Ben, and they had a charming son the same age as one of my sons. To bond us even more tightly, she and her husband were both big-time motorcycle enthusiasts.

Friday morning Dana and I decided to make one last-ditch effort to surgically develop a way to repeatedly evacuate the mucous material that her disease was producing. We hoped she could then get some relief from her pressure-related symptoms of abdominal distention and the unrelenting nausea that wasn't being controlled with any anti-emetic protocol we could come up with. Unfortunately, I wasn't able to accomplish much in the operating room, and now we had to deal with the issue of what Dana would want to do.

I had made a promise to Dana, as I do to all of my patients, that if the time came when her disease was not curable and there was really nothing more that we could do that had a legitimate chance of helping prolong her life in a meaningful way, I would tell her (and any family members she wanted me to), so that her personal preferences would be preeminent in her decision-making process. When I left the operating room, I met with Dana's husband. During our forty-five minutes together, I shared with Ben the findings of the surgery and the reality that we had run out of treatment options. He and I discussed the need to make sure that everyone who needed to be involved was fully informed about what was going on and was supportive of letting Dana make her own self-directed but data-based decisions.

The time Ben and I spent together while Dana was settling into the recovery room was accompanied by two sets of wet eyes. This number grew to three sets when I had a similar discussion with Dana and Ben in Dana's room later that evening. We talked about what was going on, and Dana asked informed and specific questions, which I answered to the best of my ability. There was much else that we shared, and the process of making end-of-life decisions went from a general "This is what I want" to a very specific "These are the issues I am facing today and tomorrow (and I hope the day beyond this), and this is exactly what I want done and why."

The biggest end-of-life decisions are the decisions regarding what an individual wants to do with the time she or he has left and where and with whom the person wants to spend that time. Before people can make decisions about what they want to do with the end of their lives, however, they need to be fully aware and understand that they are coming to the end of their lives. This statement may sound ridiculous, but recent scientific investigations have shown that we health care professionals are not as forthright and open with our patients (all of whom have placed their trust in us that we will be honest) as we should be in sharing with them the truth about their disease and life expectancy.

Though some of this "failure to disclose" is a response to an expressed or implied "failure to want to know" (that is, the patient tells the health care provider or otherwise lets the provider know that he or she does not want to know the truth), much of it is a result of the emotional pain that health care professionals feel when they have to confess, first to themselves, and then to the patient, that neither of them is going to get the preferred outcome (semipermanent reestablishment of patient wellness).

We find it extremely hard to tell someone that she is going to die and that we (and the body of scientific knowledge and the health system that we represent) have failed her. We share our inner emotions and feelings of inadequacy at not being able to facilitate the "saving of a life" with only a very small percentage of our patients, but we tell almost all of our patients how much it means to us that they trust us with their lives. As Rick has said in the past (and as was captured on camera and then broadcast on the television documentary *Hopkins 24/7*), it never ceases to amaze him how young women who are dying will try to make *him* feel better when he confesses to them that he believes he has failed them.

What Do You Want to Do with the Time You Have Left?

Rick says, "I ask my patients this question point blank. I need to relieve my own conscience that I have brought the issue up and that they have heard this from me." Do you want to spend your time being treated with therapies that have a very low rate of response but a well-known, predictable, and documented rate of toxicity? Do you want to take a trip, go visit someone, accomplish something special? Is there a unique event that you want so much to attend you are willing to try almost anything to make it to the event? A wedding, a Bar Mitzvah, the birth of grandchild, or something similar?

Part of the answer to this question involves a person's attitude toward "going gently into that good night." The range of attitudes in this regard is truly remarkable. The following is an example from Rob's practice:

Rob recently had a patient whose disease recurred quickly. The patient was re-operated on and repeatedly re-treated. No matter what was done, the disease just kept growing, and the future and the time line had become certain. Despite significant persistent side effects of her treatments, which were added to the effects of progressive disease, she just wanted to keep going at it. We were running out of drugs to use, a situation that is very uncommon. This patient eventually died from a combination of progressive disease and toxicity of treatment. But to the end she was asking for more. And what was uniquely amazing about this exemplary woman was not that she wanted to keep going at life—something we often see in young women who have many life challenges and tasks ahead of them—but that she was approaching the average age of death for American women. Although she was interested in seeing a new grandchild born, that wasn't the real motivator. What motivated her was simply a personal code that she was "never going to give up."

Of course, this is an unusual case. More commonly, women decide they have reached a point where they have had enough and they just want to be left alone. They want quality, not quantity, and are willing to do a lot to get that quality.

One of our "rules to practice by" on the Kelly Gynecologic Oncology Service at the Johns Hopkins Hospital and Medical Institutions is never to assume how a patient will answer a question. This credo should be applied to *every* decision, whether active or by default, that a patient can make, but it is never more crucial in the natural history of a woman with ovarian cancer than when she is making end-of-life decisions. Every change in medication, every new blood test ordered, every visit that is scheduled, must be done in association with the patient's verbal confirmation that "This is what I want done." When there is little time left, it is incredibly important that every minute be spent in a way that is completely consistent with the patient's wishes.

Where and with Whom Do You Want to Spend the Time You Have Left?

Several specific questions need to be considered by patients who are facing the end of life.

Where Do You Want to Die? With the wide availability of home hospice in the United States, there is no reason a patient can't receive all of her health care and services to relieve suffering at home—services that until the 1980s were generally only available in the inpatient setting. So from the perspective of quality of life, there should no difference between spending one's last days at home or in a hospital. In all honesty, however, this lack of difference exists only in an ideal world. In the real world, where there are insurance and resource limitations, it may be difficult for a given individual to receive the same care at home as in a hospital. This should not be the case, but unfortunately it often is.

There are, of course, many people who don't want to die at home. Certain religious traditions have taboos about the spirits of dead individuals and where they are released when the body dies. Some patients do not want family members to bear the memory of a dead body in the house. And there are other reasons why a person may not want to die in her home or in the home of a friend or family member. Whether *we* find the reasons rational doesn't matter: to the patient, these reasons are real and valid. We need to respect the reasons fully and help the patient spend her last days where she chooses, if at all possible.

How Alert Do You Want to Be? Though one of the goals of optimal pain relief is to relieve pain to the greatest degree possible while maintaining functionality, there are some times, as death approaches, when there is a trade-off between total pain control and total alertness. Some patients are willing to deal with low or even moderate degrees of pain if doing so means they can have maximum alertness. For some individuals, even the slightest amount of pain is too much; they might say that if eliminating all pain means some sleepiness and lack of ability to be attentive, so be it. Health care providers need to address these issues and have an open and frank discussion leading to an understanding with the patient.

Do You Want to Be Intubated or to Have Cardiopulmonary Resuscitation (CPR)? This question would only come into consideration if the patient "coded" (short for *Code Blue,* the traditional voice page that used to be called when a patient stopped breathing or lost a pulse or blood pressure). The implied obligation of a health care professional in this situation, unless explicitly informed otherwise, is to keep a patient "alive" until even the most heroic efforts have failed.

It was demonstrated in the 1980s that when people with a terminal disease process "code," few of them leave the intensive care unit alive. Also, a person who is in the intensive care unit (where she must be if she is intubated and on a ventilator or is receiving certain medications) is physically isolated from those individuals who matter to her most. Even if a patient has chosen to die at home, she is not protected from being taken to the hospital and intubated and aggressively resuscitated, unless she provides specific instructions to the contrary. An example:

> One Sunday evening when Rick was covering the Kelly Gynecologic Oncology Service, he received a call from the daughter of one of his partner's patients, Marion S., who had decided to die at home. The daughter described to Rick the pattern of her mother's breathing and said that her mom was not very responsive. The daughter wanted to know what she should do. Even though Marion had explicitly stated her desire to die at home and not to undergo heroic attempts at resuscitation, and had made this clear to her daughter and family, if the daughter had called 911, the paramedics would have performed CPR and transferred Marion to the nearest hospital unless there was a written and valid "Do not resuscitate" order.

Understandably, Marion's daughter was scared. Rick spent a few minutes going over the issues with her and summarizing both her mother's wishes and what might happen over the next few hours. Fortunately, Marion fell deeper into sleep and literally passed to the beyond in her home, with the person she loved the most in the whole world (and who in return loved Marion the most) at her side.

There are many ways of making sure that an individual's wishes regarding heroic measures are respected. Probably the best way is to execute a *living will,* which is a legal instrument that explicitly states what an individual wants done (and does not want done) at the end of life. We strongly encourage every one of our patients to complete one of these documents and have it notarized, and then to give copies of the document to family members, friends, health care professionals, lawyers, and so on. The more people who have copies of the living will, the better the situation.

Another legal instrument, similar but distinctly different, is the *durable power of attorney for health care.* In this legal document, people designate the individual or individuals who will serve as a surrogate for them, making health care decisions for them if they are unable to do so. The durable power of attorney for health care does not specify what is going to be done; it only designates who is going to make the decisions about what will be done if the patient cannot. Rick says, "Both Kate and I have living wills and durable powers of attorney for health care. We have designated each other as surrogates, and we have named alternates (friends, brothers, and so forth), as well. Interestingly, our living wills are different as to what we want done . . . but that is another story altogether!"

What Do You Want Done with Your Mortal Remains? What Kind of Funeral or Wake or Party or Ceremony Do You Want to Take Place after You Die? This decision can be made at any time during one's life and therefore is not necessarily an end-of-life decision, but it becomes increasingly timely as one comes closer to death. Here's a personal example that Rick offers:

> One of the most interesting discussions I ever had with my parents occurred in the business-class cabin of a US Airways airplane between Philadelphia and Munich one fall. I like to take trips with my parents every year or two, serving as part tour guide, part caregiver. One fall they wanted to go back to Italy, where they had lived for a couple of years in their early twenties shortly after World War II. We flew together, my parents sitting beside each other and I in the seat behind. After we were "at our cruising altitude" and the pilot had turned off the "fasten seat belt sign," I moved up and sat on the floor in front of my parents. We were just chitchatting, and the fact came up that these seventy-eight-year-olds had both visited the mortician to make decisions regarding what they wanted done if they should die. With a little prodding, they shared their decisions.
>
> My Mom wanted to be cremated, have her ashes put in a nice urn (the cheapest one the mortician showed them was 500 bucks!), and have a nice memorial service (funeral) in her local church followed by a "lunch." My Dad also wanted to be cremated, though he didn't want to spend the money on the urn (we decided that a Folgers pound-and-a-half coffee can would work nicely . . . Thanks, Cohen brothers), wasn't into the church and reception thing, and agreed that the family could go out to dinner together afterward but that I had to pay for it and the cost couldn't be charged against his estate. He wanted his ashes spread across the prairies and upper Missouri river, an area where he has lived for more than forty-seven years. Because my parents thought about what they want and shared their wishes with me (my Mom actually wrote hers down and noted what songs she wanted to be sung and what readings she was interested in), I can do my best to make sure that their wishes are respected.

Just as with the living will and the durable power of attorney for health care, it is a good idea to decide whether you have any strongly held wishes about funerals, body management, flowers, and other details. Write your wishes down and tell the people you trust about them.

Chapter 13

Death and the Process of Dealing with Loss

When is a person dead? Although the legal system has given us code after code as a result of difficult tort cases, the definition of death still seems elusive. Rick recounts a couple of stories to inform our reflections:

My Mom's dad had multiple medical problems before he died. He had a primary gastric cancer (I still remember being in the patient waiting area at St. Luke's Hospital in Cedar Rapids, Iowa, when we visited him as he recovered from his subtotal gastrectomy). However, being of tough immigrant Nordic-Deutsch stock, his body wouldn't give up yet. Unfortunately, he was severely impaired both mentally and physically as a result of multiple strokes. The last eighteen or so months of his life were spent receiving full-time "nursing" care in his home, supplied by his wife of almost sixty years, my grandmother Emma Meier Stolte. During that time there really didn't appear to be much left of that incredibly strong Germanic farmer other than a frail and marginally functional body.

Grandpa Stolte died when I was sixteen and was unquestionably still developing my own personal worldview (still am, my wife, Kate, would say). When my grandfather died, my grandmother didn't outwardly show much sign of loss. I remember her commenting on that very fact in my presence. What she said has stuck with me: "Emil died when he was no

longer able to communicate with me. I did most of my griev-
ing then."

A few days ago I was walking outside between buildings at
the Johns Hopkins Hospital and Medical Institutions cam-
pus (as I like to do, to avoid staying inside the hospital buildings and blasting down hallways full of processed air), returning to my academic office from the Weinberg Building,
having completed my second of three major surgeries for the
day. I was tumbling over in my mind all the issues I was dealing with at that time, but mostly weighing family closeness
against career. Out of nowhere, my grandfather Montz
(known as Doc) was with me. Something had made me remember him, and think about his unyielding commitment to
just and high-quality patient care. I felt that if I had wanted
to, I could have picked up a phone and called him to ask his
sage (and quite opinionated and probably profane) advice. Although Doc had been physically dead for twenty-three years,
longer than I have been a doctor, he was very, very alive.

These two stories (without even mentioning the Christian
concept of eternal life) touch on the question "When are we
dead?" In more spiritual and humanistic realms, the answer
might be "It depends."

By legal and medical statute and convention, death occurs
at the moment when there is no longer measurable cardiac activity. In a setting away from health facilities or cardiac monitoring, this is said to be the time when there is no longer a detectable pulse or heart pumping. If monitoring is occurring, a
person is considered to be dead when there is no longer measurable cardiac electric activity on a monitor (electrocardiogram).

There is some value in understanding the concept of *brain
death*, the situation in which the person has cardiopulmonary
function (as a result of either natural function or artificial support) but a series of accepted tests have demonstrated that the
brain is not working at all, even on a reflexive basis. Tests to determine brain death are usually done so that artificial support

of cardiac or pulmonary function can be removed. Of course, patients need to be in the hospital to receive this support (usually an intensive care unit, or ICU), and it is there that a decision is made whether to continue what would be considered futile efforts.

In fifteen years as an attending gynecologic oncologist, Rick remembers only two instances when it was necessary to make a determination about brain death so as to withdraw cardiopulmonary support. Neither of these women had a malignancy, but both had suffered "codes" and had been through a long period during which their brains didn't get much or any oxygen. A strict protocol for determining brain death (which had been developed by the medical faculty and approved by both the legal office and the ethics committee of the institutions where he was practicing) was followed before pulmonary support was withdrawn. Withdrawing pulmonary support means stopping the respirator that is keeping the lungs working and is causing oxygen to go into the blood of the patients; this action is sometimes called "pulling the plug," a term that comes from the idea of stopping the electricity that runs through the mechanical ventilator. After the respirator was stopped, the tube in the patient's throat was gently removed. Cardiac monitoring continued until all electrical activity stopped, something that took only a few moments in both of the cases. These patients, whom Rick had cared for and cared about, were now dead.

Why does death frighten us so much? For most modern people who do not hold any of the traditional medieval beliefs about a physical purgatory or hell, psychologists tell us that the fear of death is not fear of what is on "the other side," but concerns about losing something valuable and about what will happen to those we care about once we are gone. Many of our patients, having accomplished all that they had hoped for in their lives, and seeing the people and things that mattered most to them either precede them in death or lose meaning, have looked forward to death, even longed for it. They had nothing to lose, nothing to worry about, and were anxious to "get on." Most often these are older people, and many have just recently lost a long-

time life mate. We all know of examples of these couples. Recently an individual who was a major influence in Rick's life was
in this situation:

> Burt N. was my high school civics teacher. He was a great guy,
> trying to make the most out of what was mostly a group of
> marginally talented and motivated kids. Burt always did it in
> a respectful way and often taught some simple though in-
> credibly valuable lessons along the way. I will never forget a
> sign he hung in his office. It said: "If you think that you are
> irreplaceable, just put your fist into a bucket of water and
> then pull it out. You are as difficult to replace as it was to fill
> the hole left in the water when you removed your hand." That
> one has stayed with me.
>
> Burt and his wife had been married more than fifty years,
> had raised five kids, and had seen them all move out of the
> state. As they got into their late seventies, they sold their
> house and moved into an assisted living complex close to my
> parents. Though both were in good health for folks of their
> age, Burt got a bad cold and quickly died. Six weeks later his
> life mate, who had nothing physically wrong with her, was
> gone too. She had lived her life and had had enough. In some
> metaphysical way I know that these two individuals, who at
> least outwardly appeared to be so tightly bound to each other,
> are together.

Most of the women who are our patients are not at a place
in their lives where they are willing to stop living. Many have resolved issues of loss and separation, but few desire death. Rick
and his wife had a relevant experience:

> Kate once underwent an evaluation and was noted to have an
> X-ray finding that was suspicious for the presence of an ag-
> gressive form of uterine cancer. A diagnostic procedure
> needed to be performed to determine whether a malignancy
> was present. As the day of the procedure came closer and

closer, Kate became less anxious as I became more. What had happened? Well, Kate had made me promise that, if something happened to her, I would give up my seventy-hour-a-week work style plus frequent travel, and focus on the care of our kids. Once I had unhesitatingly agreed to do just that, Kate, knowing that my conscience would make me keep my word, had less concern about what would happen to those she would leave and was more comfortable with the future. I, on the other hand, realized that I could potentially be losing two of the three most valued "things" in my life: my soulmate life partner and my mission-driven career. I feared the unknown and the loss of something that was immeasurably valuable. Happily, no cancer was present, Kate was successfully treated, and normality was reestablished.

This vignette illustrates a point: it is the loss of that which we value that makes death frightening.

Death is something that cancer doctors must become accustomed to but should never become comfortable with. If the death of one of our patients fails to sadden us, we have lost that critical gift of caring that made us worthy of being labeled doctors (and the same goes for nurses). Caring for dying people must always be painful; it can never become routine. Every time one of our patients dies, no matter how close or distant our emotional attachment is to him or her, a small part of us dies as well. It is one of those great mysteries of the human spirit that we can repeatedly die yet still have more to give. This miracle falls into that category which includes a parent's endless love and a soldier's endless courage.

As we discussed in the Chapter 12, we encourage our patients, even when they are fighting their hardest to live, to reflect upon their death. Where do they want to be? Who do they want to be with? What do they want to happen afterward regarding donation of body parts, cremation or burial, memorial services and "celebrations of life"? Who do they want to inherit whatever temporal possessions or resources they have? Who do they want to take over for them (not replace them!) in their roles in the family and community? Even thinking about these issues can be paralyzingly painful for some women. However, these issues really must be addressed.

Elisabeth Kübler-Ross, in her landmark book *On Death and Dying*, describes how dealing with loss is a process. The process of dealing with loss is as important as reaching the end goal of acceptance of loss.

Most individuals require professional help in dealing with the concepts of loss and death. We strongly encourage our patients, early in their disease process, to develop a relationship with an individual or individuals who can help them through the process of coping with the idea of their own death. This person may be a pastor, priest or rabbi, a psychologist, a social worker, or a counselor. Support group therapy (such as the therapy available at Wellness Communities) often can be helpful. Taking an active approach, at the woman's own pace and with support from others, makes it likely that the woman will be prepared if she faces death. We hope that death will not be the eventual outcome of ovarian cancer. However, should it be, the woman will be best prepared if the issues surrounding the end of life and death have been addressed and processed.

Chapter 14

Survivorship

If it is relatively easy, within the limitations we have discussed, to define when one dies, shouldn't it be easy to define when one is surviving? Well, guess what? It isn't. If you define surviving using purely biological criteria, well, then, yes, surviving is not being dead. But surviving is so much more than that! Ideally, it is being intellectually, spiritually, and physically fully functional. And we love to aim for the ideal.

As we pointed out earlier in this book, the stress of the diagnosis and treatment of ovarian cancer can push marginally functional relationships over the edge. The same holds true for everything we are and do. A person may be willing to put up with a barely acceptable job, for example, until she literally looks death in the eye, realizes that life is a very limited commodity, and says, "Take this job and shove it"—to quote the old country and western song. What about interpersonal relationships? How she spends her leisure time? What she does with money? And on and on . . .

Dealing with ovarian cancer can remarkably change what a person is satisfied with and how she wants to live her life. It actually allows—or forces—individuals to address issues they have never addressed before. We have seen many women come out on the other side of their initial cancer treatment happier and more fulfilled than when they entered, because they had decided that taking stock of their lives and actively managing them was essential. (See the story of Inez V., below.) Unfortunately,

women can also come out on the other side of their initial ovarian cancer treatment a total emotional, intellectual, and physical wreck, paralyzed by fear as to when the cancer was going to
come back and angry at everyone about everything. Here are two
stories. One is a story of how not to survive; the other is a story
of how to survive.

Isabel P. was diagnosed with ovarian cancer in her early seventies and underwent all the appropriate therapies. Fortunately, she fell into that group of ladies whose disease goes
into remission. But she was suffering more after her treatment than she ever did before. She was angry at God for having done this to her. She had decided to leave her long-term
home and move closer to where her children lived . . . and she
hated her new home. She said she didn't have any friends,
didn't like the weather, and so on. And even though she had
regained her strength, she couldn't sleep at night because she
was so afraid the cancer would come back. She said there
were days when she just wished she was dead (a professional
mental health worker called in by Isabel's doctor determined
that Isabel did not pose a risk to herself). Isabel P. was *not surviving,* although she was very much alive and would be for a
significant time to come, barring an accident or sudden death
from some other medical problem.

Inez V., too, was diagnosed with ovarian cancer and had all
the standard therapies. Her story is similar to Isabel P.'s,
except for one factor: Inez's disease recurred about five
months after she completed initial therapy. Not long after
that, her life partner of eighteen years died of a heart attack.
Yet Inez decided that she was going to listen to the wake-up
call she had received from the ovarian cancer. She was going
to control her life and try to be as happy as possible for as long
as possible. She joined a yoga program at the local Wellness
Community, started water-color painting (something she had
been doing on and off her whole life but had let slip to the

sidelines while she was raising her children and working), and was enjoying lunching with friends (though in a modest way, since, she confessed, her retirement benefits were limited). She joyfully painted a wonderful still life that hangs in the director's conference room of our department. Inez V. realizes that her life is short, and though she is sad when she thinks that she will likely die before her grandkids graduate from college or marry—events she had hoped to attend—she is grateful for every day she has and for the limited nature of the suffering she has experienced to date.

Which of these two ladies is surviving? We would suggest that Inez V., who is actively dying, is the one who is surviving, while Isabel P., who has no physical, chemical, or radioactive evidence of disease, is not surviving.

Really, it has to do with how you define *survivorship*. We discussed some of these issues in Chapter 13, but there is value in reviewing them. Life is a terminal disease process, and we all will eventually physically die. And though there are lots of folks who believe and who will tell you that there is an "eternal life," few Americans believe that this eternal life is going to be much like what our everyday lives are like. Therefore, most of us believe that when you die, you (that physical you that can be described in height, weight, and hair and eye color, but also the personality you) are not going to exist in any way that resembles the you whom your family and friends know. For the people we know as ourselves, this time may well be the only time around.

But what about life, and survivorship? Just having a heartbeat and breathing, or even having cognitive thought, may on a certain level constitute life, but they don't define *survival*. Survival is finding joy in the world around us, even when our lives are not necessarily the way we want them to be. Being productive and useful, even when we may not be able to do all that we used to be able to do or all that we could have done. Having a meaning and serving a purpose for others. That is survivorship!

Since September 2001, many pundits have talked about how much of the financial and moral degeneration that has occurred is really our own fault. We Americans, they claim, have become very "me focused." What is in it *for me?* How can I get ahead— get more money, possessions, fame, power? Sadly, generation after generation and life story after life story have demonstrated that when we focus on what is measurable (bank account balances, number of cars, cost of the latest piece of clothing) rather than on what is immeasurable (who cares for us and whom do we care for? how much are we putting back into the community?), we are condemned to be unhappy, because we are never going to be able to get enough. Remember that old appellation "poor little rich girl"?

Being alive is having meaning and making a difference. Let's answer this question: If an individual is totally isolated from the rest of the world, never, ever interacting in any way and having absolutely no impact on anyone else's life, so that no one knows that she or he exists, *does* she or he exist?

No one can argue that the personality we were born with makes no difference in how we view our situation, how good or bad we consider our lives to be. Different patients will respond differently to the diagnosis and treatment of ovarian cancer because they have different personalities. What we are talking about in this chapter, however, is our desire to help our patients toward survivorship, even taking personality differences into account.

When a patient of ours is having difficulty finding any pleasure in life (a condition called *anhedonia*), we, as health care professionals, must first take steps to find out whether she is clinically depressed. One who is depressed might respond very well to having focused care from an experienced mental health provider. If the patient is not depressed but still is having a difficult time of it, we try to counsel her, talking about some of the ideas in this chapter.

It is most important to recognize where the "comfort zone" of survivorship is for you as an individual. Not everyone can be as proactive and engaged in life as Inez V.; however, no one should suffer as much and be as disconnected from life as Isabel P. Ovarian cancer is a traumatizing illness, no question about it. It is an illness that requires treatment not only of the cancer, but of the whole person as well. True survivorship is something that can be defined only by you, as you consider your unique personal feelings and life goals. Recognizing that you are out of your comfort zone, and allowing your doctor and other health care professionals, family and friends, or clergy to help, can be the first steps toward really "surviving" ovarian cancer.

Each woman diagnosed with ovarian cancer will have her own, very personal definition of survivorship, and the particulars of how she navigates that journey are equally unique to her as an individual. In general terms, however, a large component of "surviving" ovarian cancer has to do with being in control of one's life as much as possible and being as "well" (in all aspects of Wellness) as possible, and with finding joy and pleasure in living life to the fullest extent possible. This book is not intended to be an instruction book that will work for everyone. Instead, we provide it as a guide, a resource to help patients define their own path to surviving ovarian cancer and beyond.

Resources

American Cancer Society, Inc.
(ACS)
1599 Clifton Road, NE
Atlanta, GA 30329
1-800-ACS-2345
www.cancer.org

American Society of Clinical
Oncology (ASCO)
1900 Duke Street, Suite 200
Alexandria, VA 22312
703-299-0150
www.oncology.com

Cancer Care, Inc.
275 Seventh Avenue
New York, NY 10001
212-302-2400
1-800-813-HOPE
www.cancercare.org

Gilda Radner Familial Ovarian
Cancer Registry
Elm and Carlton Streets
Buffalo, NY 14263
1-800 OVARIAN
www.ovariancancer.com

Gilda's Club
322 Eighth Avenue, Suite 1402
New York, NY 10001
1-800-GILDA4U
www.gildasclub.org

Look Good . . . Feel Better
1101 17th Street NW, Suite 300
Washington, DC 20036-4702
1-800-395-LOOK
www.lookgoodfeelbetter.org

National Cancer Institute (NCI)
1-800-4-Cancer
www.nci.nih.gov
www.cancer.gov/cancerinfo/coping

National Coalition for Cancer
Survivorship
1010 Wayne Avenue, Suite 770
Silver Spring, MD 20910-5600
877-622-7937
www.canceradvocacy.org

National Ovarian Cancer
Association (NOCA)
416-962-2700
www.ovariancanada.org

The National Ovarian Cancer
Coalition, Inc. (NOCC)
500 NE Spanish River Boulevard,
Suite 8
Boca Raton, FL 33431
1-888-OVARIAN
NOCC@ovarian.com
www.ovarian.org

The Neuropathy Association
www.neuropathy.org
Oncology Nursing Society
www.ons.org

The Ovarian Cancer Connection
P.O. Box 7948
Amarillo, TX 79114-7948
806-355-2565
*Conversations! The International
Newsletter for Those Fighting
Ovarian Cancer*
chmelancon@aol.com
www.ovarian-news.com

Ovarian Cancer National Alliance
910 17th Street NW, Suite 413
Washington, DC 20006
202-331-1332
www.ovariancancer.org

Ovarian Cancer Research Fund,
Inc. (OCRF)
1-800-873-9569
www.ocrf.org

Patient Advocate Foundation
(PAF)
1-800-532-5274
www.patientadvocate.org

SHARE: Self-Help for Women
with Breast or Ovarian Cancer
212-719-0364
866-891-2392
www.sharecancersupport.org

Society of Gynecologic
Oncologists
401 N. Michigan Avenue
Chicago, IL 60611
1-800-444-4441
www.sgo.org

The Wellness Community
919 18th Street NW, Suite 54
Washington, DC 20006
www.thewellnesscommunity.org

Women's Cancer Network
1-800-444-4441
www.wcn.org

Index

About the Authors

Fredrick J. "Rick" Montz was born in Marshfield, Wisconsin, in 1955. His professional accomplishments are overshadowed only by the vigor with which he embraced all that life had to offer prior to his unexpected and premature death in 2002. Rick received his Bachelor of Arts degree from Concordia College in Moorhead, Minnesota, and his medical degree from Baylor College of Medicine in Houston, Texas. After residency in obstetrics and gynecology at the University of Southern California Medical Center in Los Angeles, he completed fellowships at St. George's Hospital, University of London School of Medicine in England, and at the University of Southern California Norris Cancer Center in Los Angeles. He joined the faculty at the University of California, Los Angeles, School of Medicine in 1987 and a decade later was recruited to the Johns Hopkins University School of Medicine, where he achieved the rank of Professor of Gynecology, Obstetrics, Oncology, and Surgery while serving as Director of the Kelly Gynecologic Oncology Service at the Johns Hopkins Hospital. Rick was a consummate physician, researcher, teacher, mentor, and colleague renowned at Hopkins and nationwide for his extraordinary and boundless ability to communicate with and comfort the thousands who sought his care. He was a loving and devoted husband and father and considered his family the source of all that was peaceful, joyous, and life-affirming.

Robert E. Bristow received his Bachelor of Arts degree from Pomona College in Claremont, California, and his medical degree from the University of Southern California Medical Center in Los Angeles. After completing his residency in gynecology and obstetrics at the Johns Hopkins University School of Medicine, he received his fellowship training in gynecologic oncology at the University of California, Los Angeles, School of Medicine. In 1998 Dr. Bristow returned to Johns Hopkins, where he is currently Associate Professor of Gynecology, Obstetrics, and Oncology and Director of the Kelly Gynecologic Oncology Service at the Johns Hopkins Hospital. He is the author of numerous scientific publications regarding women's cancer, with a particular focus on improving the care for women with ovarian cancer.

Paula J. Anastasia has been an oncology nurse for twenty years. She received her Bachelor of Arts and Bachelor of Science in Nursing from Rush University in Chicago, and her Master's of Nursing from the University of California, Los Angeles. She worked collaboratively with Drs. Montz and Bristow at UCLA and is currently the gynecologic-oncology clinical nurse specialist at Cedars-Sinai in Los Angeles, where she coordinates the management of gynecologic oncology patients in the outpatient setting with surgical, chemotherapy, and radiation therapy. She is actively involved in her local Oncology Nursing Society Chapter, the Wellness Community, and the American Cancer Society. Her clinical passion is caring for women with ovarian cancer, with an emphasis on managing their symptoms and improving their quality of life.